"Chung crafts a deeply personal reckoning with our country's entrenched inequalities and an elegy for her parents . . . and provides a rare record of the difficulty of supporting a parent through end-of-life care. . . . *A Living Remedy* provides a powerful remembrance and a path forward."
—NPR

"*A Living Remedy* is a bouquet of feeling—Nicole Chung weaves a groundbreaking narrative steeped in love, humor, the infinitude of memory, and the essentiality of community. Chung approaches the kaleidoscope of grief from its many angles, excavating its complexity with heart and candor. But Chung's prose also soothes, uncovering hidden corners of the heart and its many permutations. *A Living Remedy* is elegiac and heart-expanding, a memoir that's both an exploration of loss and a beacon for moving forward. We couldn't be luckier to have this gift of a book."
—BRYAN WASHINGTON, AUTHOR OF *Memorial*

"*A Living Remedy* is a profoundly moving account of one daughter's love for her white adoptive parents and a damning indictment of the health-care system that failed them. Nicole Chung writes with nuance and empathy about what it means to be ill and economically insecure in America today. She transforms her rage and anguish into luminous prose on the page, and the result is one of the most devastating portraits of a daughter's grief I have ever read."
—JULIE OTSUKA, AUTHOR OF *The Swimmers*

"This riveting and tender memoir is a stunning meditation on grief and guilt, driven by the ways in which the U.S. health-care system, one of the highest costs of health care in the world, fails those that cannot afford it. Detailing her father's inability to access health care and his premature death, Chung illuminates the hardships many Americans face caring for aging parents and loved ones in a broken system."
—LUPITA AQUINO, TODAY.COM

"This openhearted, unflinching account will be a boon to others."
—*Kirkus Reviews*

"*A Living Remedy* is a book about love, loss, leaving home, and finding home. Nicole Chung has a rare, precious gift: the ability to tell an intimate story with vast social implications. *A Living Remedy* is a book that honors the way families are made through a collage of close encounters and shared struggles. Brimming with insight about class, race, identity, and politics, it will move and transform readers with its beauty, spirituality, and wisdom." —IMANI PERRY, AUTHOR OF *South to America*

"This fiery book combines a chronicle of the grief of losing one's parents and a searing indictment of the unequal health-care system that led to their early deaths." —*People*

"A delicate, painful, magnificent book." —*Elle*

"This astounding and immensely moving memoir is a gift. It is a chance to think about family, mortality, love, and grief. It is a chance to confront the broken health-care system we live within. From the most intimate to the most public, *A Living Remedy* holds gemlike questions about all that matters." —MEGHA MAJUMDAR, AUTHOR OF *A Burning*

"On one level, Nicole Chung's second memoir is an elegy for her adoptive parents. On another, it's an indictment of the broken health-care systems that prevent a disappearing middle class from receiving the affordable care they desperately need." —*Harper's Bazaar*

"*A Living Remedy* stands to spark a major and essential conversation. . . . Chung excels at excavating both the personal and the systemic." —LITERARY HUB

"Chung applies the same incisive intimacy with which she explored her reconnection with her birth family in her first book to examine her profound relationships with her white adoptive parents. . . . Chung's prose hones her grief into razor-sharp insights even as her words interrogate, honor, and celebrate the unbreakable bonds of parenthood." —*Booklist* (STARRED REVIEW)

"An unforgettable, transformative read. Nicole Chung shows the deep pits of grief and the messy reality of life after loss, revealing pain, financial insecurity, and the failures of our country's health-care system with tender lucidity. This is a profound memoir that haunted and nourished me. I cried. I ached. I saw a path forward."

—CRYSTAL HANA KIM, AUTHOR OF *If You Leave Me*

"As Chung immerses readers in her experience of grief, her powerful words compel us to follow her on a beautiful but difficult journey of loss. . . . *A Living Remedy* makes this era of collective grief more personal, as Chung honestly explores her childhood and the lives and deaths of her parents. She gives these hard times a purpose, absorbing them with both fury and compassion, making them part of her own legacy to pass along to her daughters. For her, this is indeed a living remedy."

—*BookPage* (STARRED REVIEW)

"A visceral and wrenching memoir."

—*Esquire*

"This narrative investigates grief and unequal access to health care as much as it does the love that makes a family whole."

—*Boston Globe*

"Searing. . . . A poignant book that's sure to resonate widely."

—*Parade*

A LIVING
REMEDY

A LIVING

REMEDY

A Memoir

NICOLE

CHUNG

An Imprint of HarperCollins*Publishers*

FIRST ECCO PAPERBACK EDITION PUBLISHED 2024

Library of Congress Cataloging-in-Publication Data has been applied for.

ISBN 978-0-06-303162-3 (pbk.)

24 25 26 27 28 LBC 5 4 3 2 1

For my parents

I don't know if I'll ever go home again.
I don't know who I've seen for the last time.

—SAFIA ELHILLO, *"For My Friends, in Reply to a Question"*

What it must be like to be an angel
or a squirrel, we can imagine sooner.

—WILLIAM MEREDITH, *"Parents"*

. . . because even grief provides a living remedy

—MARIE HOWE, *"For Three Days"*

A LIVING
REMEDY

1

I CAN PICTURE HER, ONE PALE, FRECKLED CHEEK RESTING
on the yellow floral-patterned pillowcase next to mine, warm
brown eyes half-lidded with sleep as she listened to me talk.
She was often tired in those days; after walking in the door,
she would greet me, drop her purse on a chair, and then go
lie down for a while before dinner. Sometimes I'd follow her
down the brown-carpeted hallway to my parents' room, the
second door on the right, directly across from mine, and chat-
ter at her from the doorway or my dad's side of the bed. She
would respond now and then, ask me the occasional question. If she fell asleep, I'd tiptoe away.

When I was little, we would sit side by side on her bed
while she told me stories about her girlhood, taught me my
prayers, got me started on early cross-stitch and crochet
projects, read me stories she loved: *A Little Princess*, *Anne of
Green Gables*, *Pride and Prejudice*. By the time I was a senior
in high school, I was mostly just looking to talk, to tell her
about my day: the tests I had coming up, the school musical

I wanted to try out for, plans my friends and I had made for the weekend. I probably should have known to leave her in peace. She wasn't in good health then, which I did not fully understand. No matter how exhausted she was, she never sent me away.

I wonder if she ever thought about how soon I'd be leaving as the two of us lay on the squeaky old mattress, late-afternoon sunlight filtering through the sheer brown curtains above us. I wonder if that's why she always let me gab when she got home from work, why she didn't tell me to go away and let her rest. Soon we'd no longer be sharing a roof, and she wouldn't hear much about my individual days, only the sum total of whatever I could remember after a full week of classes and papers and books and dining hall meals, on a Sunday afternoon phone call made with one of dozens of calling cards she mailed to me. We would still belong to each other, but we would come to know one another differently in separation, in parting after parting.

I didn't know what it would mean to leave, wouldn't begin to grasp it until my last night in my little blue childhood bedroom, a few months later, when I found I couldn't sleep for terror and wonder. I had spent most of my life in a small house in a small town, a Korean adoptee who knew I was loved but often felt as though I were living a life meant for someone else. Though dreams of escape had long held me in thrall, I missed my parents when I spent any considerable length of time away from them, and my mom was the person I most wanted to talk to at the end of the day. I'm sure plenty of people who knew me were surprised that such a homebody only child had set her sights on a life three thousand miles away. It would be years before I would understand that she was the one, all along, who had been preparing me to go. Who wanted me to have the choice.

I think of those late-afternoon talks with her now that I have my own children, knowing that the days of both of them falling asleep in their rooms down the hall from mine are dwindling; that a time will come when something trivial or life changing will happen to them—they will be hurt, or caught by surprise, or find that they are happier than they have ever been—and I will not be the first person they tell. That might be why I sometimes let them stay up past bedtime chatting with me or getting silly with each other, why even the brightest moments on the best of days can crack my heart wide open. But then sometimes I think, well, no matter where they go, no matter how far apart we are, maybe I will always be someone they think to call, someone they want to talk to, because my mother is far beyond my sight, beyond the reach of my voice, and not a day goes by when I don't think of something I wish I could tell her.

2

MY MOTHER COULD BARELY CARRY A TUNE, BUT SHE LOVED music, and she loved watching me sing. At choral concerts, musicals, voice recitals, I would seek and find her in the crowd, sitting somewhere toward the center of the room with her eyes fixed on me. Even if I sang with a hundred others, she would insist that she could pick out my voice. *The trick is to look at you while you sing. As long as I can see you, I can hear you.* The only performance she ever missed was the fall choir concert of my freshman year of high school, because she was at home recovering from a single mastectomy.

She was diagnosed with breast cancer a few weeks before she turned forty-four. I remember my parents' shock, which I saw in the tense lines of their faces, sensed in the guarded speech and absence of levity at home. We did not talk about my mother's illness as a family, except in terms of facts and scheduling: her surgery was this day; she would be discharged from the hospital on this day; she would stay home from work until this day. Compared with later crises that would unfold over months or years, the timeline of her first battle with cancer feels remarkably compressed, little more than a blink in my memory. She was diagnosed after finding a lump and undergoing a biopsy; the following week, she had a mastectomy; a few weeks later, she had a clean scan and was declared to be in remission. She didn't have to endure chemotherapy or radiation. She didn't lose her hair. She was lucky, the doctors said, that the tumor was found so early. She would forever refer to her reconstructed breast as her "Frankenboob."

I find it strange, now, that I cannot easily place myself back in that time, or recall everything I must have been feeling as she underwent treatment. I remember the things that filled my days because they seemed so jarringly, relentlessly *normal*: I went to school on the day my mother had surgery, and every day before and after. My father would have been the one to drive me to my concert that week, unless he was working and I got a ride from a friend. I went to the houses of families I babysat for on a rotating basis, where one especially kind parent asked about my mom and paid me more than usual; to church, where the congregation remembered my mother each week (*for those who are ill . . . let us pray to the Lord*); and to after-school club meetings, where I must have finally tried to tell some friends how worried I was, because I recall one girl snapping, *Your mom's cancer is all you talk about.*

At fourteen, I was old enough to sense that I shouldn't burden my parents with my fears when they were both so shaken, intent on facing this unexpected calamity and shouldering the bills that followed. Though my mother's cancer was her trauma first and foremost, its aftershocks reverberated through my life as well. Her illness almost loomed larger in hindsight, because the initial jolt had faded, and in its place was a new awareness of my family's vulnerability. I remember feeling less sure, less safe, as if anything could befall us now. I found it harder to relax, struggled to fall asleep at night. My greatest fear was losing my mother, my father, or both—to illness, fire, a car accident—and her cancer seemed to justify every anxiety I'd ever harbored.

She had been in remission for more than a year when we went to Mass one Sunday, as usual, and I found that I could not sing the Communion hymn. The hymn was about death and eternal life, as so many hymns are. I watched the musicians strum their guitars and sing the verses I had probably sung a hundred times, my eyes brimming. My mother sat beside me, singing every word if not every note, and all I could think was that if she had died, imagining her in heaven would be no comfort at all.

Later, I asked her why we had never talked about her cancer. She and I talked about most everything else, after all. I don't know what I expected her to say. Perhaps it wasn't fair of me to ask, even after a year. My mother was rarely cold and never aloof, so I knew it was something else that made her instantly withdraw, her expression a firmly closed door. Even before she spoke, I understood that my question was an intrusion on her hard-won peace, a knock she wasn't ready to answer.

"I don't need to talk about having cancer, Nicole," she told me. "I lived through it."

She did live through it. The breast cancer never returned.

But her illness, the first serious one of her life, was a turning point for our family, an upheaval from which there would be no lasting recovery.

Once, while visiting my parents, I asked my father what he was proudest of in life.

"You," he said.

I'd walked right into that one. "Besides me."

When he paused, I wondered if he would say something sarcastic, or tell me that he couldn't think of anything. But the answer he gave was confident, his face as serious as I'd ever seen it.

"I'm pretty proud," he said, "of getting out of Ohio."

Dad was thirteen years old when he was told that his mother's kidneys were failing. The first successful living kidney transplant had been performed a decade earlier, in 1954, but the procedure was risky and far from common. Hemodialysis treatment for patients with acute renal failure had recently become available, and a home dialysis machine was soon installed in his mother's bedroom.

His parents enjoyed entertaining, and their home in Euclid had been a gathering place for parties and family holiday celebrations. Now the household settled into a state of hushed anxiety. Their father's habitual jokes, usually made at someone else's expense, took on a hard, cutting edge. Dad, his brother, and his three sisters all quickly learned what was expected of them: They couldn't play or roughhouse after school. They couldn't invite friends over. The first hint of an argument would land all of them in trouble. *What the hell's the matter with you?* They walked themselves to school and to church on Sunday and kept the house as tidy as they could. My father's most deeply loathed chore was cleaning the dialysis machine.

His grades were never stellar—my mother used to wonder whether he had undiagnosed dyslexia—but he was a hard worker, adept at solving technical problems. He also found it easy to talk with people and make them laugh; his sense of humor, unlike his father's, was warm and rarely bitter. He won graphic arts and lithography awards for his work in his high school print shop, and by his senior year he'd secured a part-time training-with-pay job in the city printing department, where he spent fifteen hours a week generating interdepartmental memos, civic work orders, and official town correspondence for $1.49 an hour. He wasn't sure that college was for him, and was glad to learn a trade that might lead to a good career without a bachelor's degree. No business could be conducted without reams of paper, he thought—every company, every school, every town would always need printers.

His printing experience led him to a good entry-level job with American Greetings after he graduated from high school. He took a couple of night classes at the community college, where he met my mother, a first-year student hoping to become a nurse. A year his junior, she never wore makeup, had long red hair down to her waist, and was often teased for looking younger than her nineteen years. They kept running into each other at bars and parties. One night, my father, the designated driver, impulsively asked her for a kiss before she got out of his car.

They hadn't been dating for long when he learned that his mother, whose condition was steadily worsening, had finally decided to undergo a transplant. *My mom is getting a kidney*, he told my mother. *She's going to live*. It had been so long since he had been able to imagine her getting better. A year later, she would help plan my parents' wedding and dance at their reception, healthier than she had been in a decade.

Like my father, my mother was born in Cleveland, but her family had left the city when she was two. My grandmother was convinced that my grandfather, who was carrying trauma after serving in World War II, would fare better in the country, so they bought a little house on some land about twenty miles outside the city. As the second eldest of five kids, Mom had a lot of responsibility at home, but her childhood was freer than Dad's: she and her siblings were allowed to be loud and rambunctious, play pranks, hunt and fish, run through woods and farmland with their dogs. During the summer, their parents would cram them into the station wagon, and the family would camp their way from one historic site or national park to another. One year they made it all the way to Everett, Washington, to visit my grandmother's beloved aunt, and Mom fell in love with the Cascades, the pine forests, and the Salish Sea—that was where she was going to live someday, she decided.

She applied to nursing school out west shortly before she and my father got engaged, but when he was offered a job in Ketchikan, Alaska, there was no question that they would go. They spent the first two years of their marriage there before relocating to Seattle, the city of my mother's dreams, where she worked as a respiratory therapist and he decided to enter a restaurant-management certificate program. It seemed like a promising career change; my father had seen other friends move into the service industry, and they assured him that he would be great at it. A regional pizza chain soon hired him to manage one of its new locations in southern Oregon. My parents found their new home a bit quiet compared with Seattle and far less beautiful than Alaska, and did not expect to stay in the region for long. But transfers and job opportunities in Portland, Denver, and Boise didn't come through, and then my mother's parents moved into a small house across town, giving them another tether to the area—and a future child-care provider in my energetic grandmother.

In July 1981, they drove up to Seattle to adopt a ten-week-old Korean girl some friends had told them about, born severely premature to an immigrant family that did not believe they could raise a medically complex child. The doctors told my adoptive parents that I would have multiple disabilities and might never live independently, but they had spent weeks praying about the adoption and believed that I was meant to be theirs. Though they had initially wondered how their families would react to having an Asian child in the family, they stopped worrying when my grandmother charged them to *go get that baby girl and bring her home to us*. Given my history, they weren't surprised when I crawled and walked later than average; they *were* surprised that by age two I spoke in paragraphs and was able to memorize anything that was read to me. Every day was a ceaseless drumbeat of questions and observations: *why* this, *why* that, *I saw, I heard, I want to tell you, did you notice, do you think* . . . *?* A neighbor with four children jokingly told my mother that if I had been her first, she would have stopped at one.

They were still adjusting to their new life as parents when Dad's mother fell ill again, her body rejecting its foreign organ. My father took me to Cleveland to see her. In photos from that visit, I am a chubby, happy one-year-old in a flowered blouse and a blue corduroy jumper, no longer small for my age, boasting a toothy grin, chipmunk cheeks, and black hair that sticks straight up in defiance of my parents' styling efforts—no one had ever told them about Asian baby hair. My grandmother, who looks so much like my father with her wide smile, broad nose, and brown hair so dark it could almost be black like mine, reaches toward me as Dad props me up on her hospital bed. He must have known that the trip was an introduction as well as a goodbye. As grieved as he would be when his mother died a few months later, a part of him was relieved that she was finally beyond her pain.

—

When I try to picture my father as he was in my youth, healthy and strong, I see him working a busy lunch or dinner shift, wearing dark pants and a short-sleeved white dress shirt with a name tag pinned to it, chatting with customers. He managed a series of pizza restaurants for most of my childhood, and if I had no school and no one else was available to watch me, sometimes I'd go with him for part of the day. I remember following him into dark industrial kitchens in the predawn chill, watching him check and order inventory. Every now and then I would try to be helpful, wiping down tables or refilling paper-napkin dispensers. It was a special treat to snack on pizza or fries with him when he took a break, especially if he gave me quarters for the jukebox.

Dad did everything from cook and clean to serve and operate the cash register; whatever most needed doing in any given moment, that was his job. Working in a restaurant looked fun when I saw him joking with guests, an easy smile on his face, because it was his job to keep them relaxed and happy. As a child, I didn't see his exhaustion at the end of an open-to-close shift in a week when he'd had no days off. I didn't know about the abusive customers, the missed breaks and meals, the unpaid overtime and raises that never came through. Sometimes a restaurant would shut down, go bankrupt, or burn down, and he would need to scramble to find another position. I was in my thirties before my mother told me about the opportunities he had missed out on, often given to younger men without families who would be cheaper to promote and relocate. "Isn't that illegal?" I asked. My mother, who'd come by her pessimism honestly, shrugged and said, "That was always the explanation they gave him."

Anxious about infectious diseases and weary of hospital hours, Mom left respiratory-therapy work behind when I was in grade school. She worked for a few months in my middle-school cafeteria—I remember waving to her from the lunch line on my first day of seventh grade, giving her a hard time for not slipping me extra fries—and held other short-term jobs I don't remember, but was more often in an office, doing medical billing or administrative work, wearing the business-casual clothes I helped her pick out at Sears and JCPenney sales. Though we didn't have much to spare, she would later say that we "got by" in those years. She gave me a small allowance—not every month, but whenever she could—and my parents tried to keep their debt low and shunt money into savings.

Then she was diagnosed with cancer. She was only a few weeks out from her surgery when the restaurant my father worked for closed. By the time he found another job six months later, an hourly position at a fast-food restaurant that paid less than his previous job, any money my parents had managed to set aside was gone. Soon after that, my mother's company reorganized and laid her off.

Late one night in my junior year, she came into my room—Dad must have been working a closing shift—and said that she needed me to drive her to the emergency room. She sobbed through the entire ten-minute drive, doubled over in agony in the passenger seat, hands cradling her abdomen. I had never seen her in so much pain. I was afraid that she was dying. I don't know how I managed to keep control of the wheel, or how long we waited at the hospital for her to be seen, or when she was admitted, or whether my father came, or how I left her there, which I must have done, so that I could drive back to our house and wake up a few hours later for school. I know that I was home the following afternoon, doing homework, when my grandmother called and told me that I could come see my mother in the hospital.

Mom had trouble keeping her eyes open as she told me that she'd had emergency surgery to remove her uterus, ovaries, and fallopian tubes. I learned new words that day: *endometriosis*, *fibroids*, *hysterectomy*. She had been in pain for months. She never told me why she had not sought treatment earlier; there could have been any number of reasons. What I now know is that my parents' employment at the time was tenuous, and we had no health coverage.

At sixteen, seventeen, I knew that my parents had little

choice but to use credit cards in an emergency, but couldn't have said how much debt they carried. I didn't know anything about the health-care system, or that we sometimes had insurance and sometimes didn't, or that even when we did, the out-of-pocket burden made my parents more reluctant to use it. I remember feeling perplexed when I began applying to college and Mom mentioned that she would need to *figure out health insurance* for me, because most universities would not allow me to enroll without it. I couldn't understand why my future school would care about such a thing—I was young and healthy and typically went to the doctor only when I needed vaccinations or when my mother, always adept at diagnosing me, suspected that I needed antibiotics.

My parents didn't want me to worry about the family finances, which they believed were hardly a teenager's business—as I learned when I barged in on one of their late-night money arguments, asking them to keep it down so I could sleep, and my father, who had a quick hot temper when stressed, threw a Corelle serving bowl at the wall to get me to retreat. But there was only so much privacy in an eleven-hundred-square-foot house, and as an only child who had always been closely attuned to my parents, I noticed my father's dejection when he lost a job he was good at; my mother's relief—*thank you, Jesus*—the day we found five hundred dollars in an envelope taped to our front door, a gift from anonymous friends. I did not need to see past-due medical bills or be included in budgeting discussions to understand that we were well short of what we needed to be comfortable. By the time I began pestering my guidance counselor on a near-weekly basis—borrowing his college guidebooks and course catalogs, asking him for advice on how to apply for scholarships—I had sensed that we no longer lived *paycheck to paycheck*, as my mother had once told me, but emergency to emergency. What had seemed like stability proved to be a flimsy, shallow facsimile of it, a version known to so many American families, dependent on absolutely everything going right. When something went wrong, as it often did, I watched my parents push down their worry and fear and work harder.

Sometimes they would portray our situation as a cautionary tale: *This is why you're going to college.* They spoke of my future education as if it were a foregone conclusion, something I can now appreciate for the advantage it was— college was never presented to me as a luxury or an unlikely dream. And yet none of us were entirely sure how I would get there. *When our daughter came into our lives, we fully expected that we would be able to play a pivotal role in helping her pay for her college education*, my mother wrote in the required parent letter attached to one of my many scholarship applications. *Unfortunately, the best made plans often go awry. If ever someone was meant to go to college, Nicole is. To my dismay, we have nothing to offer to help her pay for it.*

———

Just as I had noticed that everyone around me was white, it didn't escape my notice that many people we knew lived in bigger houses, or had nicer cars, or went on exciting vacations my family couldn't afford. But I had everything I needed, and might not have been aware of our relative precarity at all had I not been both predisposed to pay attention and conditioned to care about what was "normal." I'd always been interested in how other people lived and moved through the world, because from a young age I understood that I existed beyond the margins of what was typical, wanted, or accepted in our insular community. To be an Asian girl in the place I grew up was an isolating experience, and I'd felt like an anomaly since the day I began hearing slurs from my second-grade classmates. White adults called me an "Asian princess" and demanded to know where I was from; white teachers got stuck on my surname and demanded to know how I'd gotten it; a white girl pushed me to tell her whether what she'd heard about Asian girls' vaginas was true; a white boy subjected me to "ching-chong" chants every day at recess. Observation and anticipation were among the first and only tools I had to defend myself, and so I was the sort of kid who was constantly on the lookout, measuring the delta between me and everyone I knew; between desire and reality; between the sense of safety and belonging I craved and what I actually felt.

I had made up my mind to leave southern Oregon years before I figured out how. "Of *course* you have to go," my on-again-off-again pediatrician told me once, laughing. "You'll never be satisfied here—or find anyone to marry, for that matter." No one, not even my mother, had ever said as much to me aloud, and it was somehow both affirming and mortifying to have my ambition and loneliness so clearly read by someone who barely knew me. I knew what I wanted, but I did not feel entitled to it. I was sure that I wasn't the most impressive student at my school. As glossy brochures began to fill our mailbox, sent from competitive universities located in distant towns and regions I knew nothing about, I asked my forbearing guidance counselor if he thought I was setting myself up for disappointment. "Some of the colleges on your list might seem like a reach now," he said, "but I do think you're right to consider them. I'm sure that at least a few will want to consider you."

Should I have been more worried about leaving my family? I was not privy to all the details of what they were facing, but I know there were signs I missed, or perhaps thought too little of, even as I scrambled to compensate. My mother was still recovering, emotionally and physically, from her surgeries. My father had his own medical issues and worked long, unpredictable hours at the restaurant. They were often unable to cook, so I learned how to make a few simple meals—meat loaf and baked potatoes, beef stew and bean soup, eggs and waffles, Stroganoff made with cream-of-mushroom soup, pasta with marinara sauce from a jar—and supplemented with fast food and TV dinners bought with money from my minimum-wage job, where I spent fifteen to twenty hours each week. The rest of what I earned went to clothes and shoes, gas for the car, the contact lenses I preferred to glasses, weekday breakfast and lunch; I knew nothing about free or reduced-price meals at school, perhaps because my family disapproved of what they considered "handouts" or perhaps because none of us ever thought to ask. I was able to cover my own SAT and AP exam and college application fees—which I should have been exempt from, though I didn't know that, either—and pay for my graduation cap and gown. One of my aunts sent me cash whenever she could and purchased the computer I needed for school.

If I'd started skipping class, if my grades had dropped, I'm sure someone at school would have checked on me or tried to speak with my parents. But I was a straight-A honors student who looked like a model-minority stereotype, and no one, including me, thought I needed help. If anyone outside my family had asked how I was doing, I would have said *fine, kind of stressed about grades, looking forward to graduation*, and I would have meant it. And yet when I came home from school or work to study, I don't remember feeling anything like the heady mix of curiosity and determination that would spur me on in college. What I remember is the fear of unraveling, a sense of quiet dread, and my mother telling me that if I didn't slow down and relax, I was going to get an ulcer. "I'll relax when I'm an adult," I told her, meaning, *I'll relax when I'm out of here*. When pressed, I might admit that I was afraid of failure, but what I was really afraid of was that nothing would change, and I would remain stuck in this place where I knew I didn't fit.

No one in my family was sure how to advise me on getting into college. But I had been asking my guidance counselor for advice for years, and my mother had also heard about a consultant who worked with local students. She might have given us a lower rate, or perhaps my parents gritted their teeth and put her bill on the credit card they hated using; however it happened, one day I found myself driving to her beautiful home on the hill. I told her that I wanted to study history and English, hiding a grimace when she suggested that I take a college-level engineering course to show admissions officers that I was "well-rounded." She added more schools to my list, explaining that it was a good idea to apply to some schools "with deep pockets," in case one of them wanted me enough to pay for everything. "Here are the words I want you to look for," she told me: "*School guarantees to meet the student's full demonstrated need.*"

The day I learned that I would be going to college was not the day I got my first acceptance, or my second, or my third. I remained in suspense until several financial aid letters arrived on the same afternoon, and I opened the envelopes with shaking hands to learn that I'd been offered what amounted to a free freshman year at three schools. I had to count the zeros several times before I could believe it. "You did it," my mother said. She tried to smile, but we both wound up crying instead.

As we celebrated, I wasn't thinking about how lonely I might feel, or how much I would miss my family. I couldn't comprehend what it would mean to attain that first foothold in a world they would be unable to follow me into. I didn't know that I would spend my early months on campus feeling as though I'd wandered into another country, surrounded by students who never had to worry about buying books or finding somewhere to go when the dorms closed for a holiday. When I was informed that the terms of my scholarship required me to send regular letters to rich donors, *Daddy-Long-Legs*-style, and attend luncheons where scholarship recipients would meet and express gratitude to our benefactors face-to-face, I didn't blink. As an adoptee, I had long known what it was to be considered lucky, and to be expected to be thankful for it.

Years later, when I described some of these rituals to a friend who also owed her education to need-based financial aid, she said dryly, "Tell me that you're a poor first-generation college student without telling me that you're a poor first-generation college student." I laughed, but my instinct was to tell her that I hadn't been poor—it wasn't a term I associated with my family, nor one my parents had ever used. If we were poor, wouldn't I have struggled more? If we were poor, wouldn't I have known? Not long after, I found my first Free Application for Federal Student Aid, carefully filled out by my mother. At seventeen, I wouldn't have paid much attention to our annual household income, or the fact that it amounted to considerably less than what my freshman year would cost. All I would have focused on was that our expected family contribution was zero.

Although many people identify as middle-of-the-road, middle-class, average Americans, there are differences between a working-class and a middle-class existence, and these differences can be far from subtle. If you grow up as I did and happen to be very fortunate, as I was, your family might sacrifice much so that you can go to college. You'll feel grateful for every subsequent opportunity you get, for the degrees and open doors and better-paying jobs (if you can find them), even as an unexpected, sometimes painful distance yawns between you and the place you came from—and many will expect you to express that gratitude, using your story or your accomplishments to attack those who weren't so lucky. But in this country, unless you attain extraordinary wealth, you will likely be unable to help your loved ones in all the ways you'd hoped. You will learn to live with the specific, hollow guilt of those who leave hardship behind, yet are unable to bring anyone else with them.

I spent my last few months before college working at the local Gap, a job to which I would occasionally return over holiday and summer breaks. As I had no retail experience, I did my best to project competence at my interview, emphasizing that I was a quick study (true) and a people person (less so). I suspect I got the position in part because the hiring manager saw my Asian face—*finally* an asset! I remember thinking, amused—as a way to signal the company's commitment to a kind of diversity that didn't exist in our town.

The job was minimum wage, anywhere from half to full time, and exactly what I'd expected: I'd punch in, affix a little blue square Gap logo pin to my shirt, work the cash register, refold T-shirts, restock the denim wall, chat with customers, chase dust bunnies around the sales floor with a giant broom, and punch out. Everyone I worked with was older, more attractive, and far better at flirting than I was; it was like being a freshman in drama club, I decided, albeit with less drama. I felt deeply, refreshingly normal in a way I'd always craved, as close as I'd ever get to being the girl next door. Best of all, I had no grades or applications to worry about, no questions about where I'd be in the fall—I was in carefree, college-bound limbo, waiting for my new life to begin.

I made liberal use of my employee discount and assembled a new wardrobe—three pairs of jeans, two pairs of nice wool-blend dress pants, cotton sweaters and oxford shirts, tank tops and T-shirts in a range of jewel tones, a short floral sundress, denim cutoffs and a cargo skirt, a red raincoat and a black trench and a navy-blue peacoat. After years of wearing whatever I'd found on sale at Fred Meyer or Penney's, I reveled in the ability to acquire so many nice new items from a brand I thought of as synonymous with the American teenager. My mother rolled her eyes every time I came home with another telltale blue shopping bag, but every purchase seemed necessary to me. These clothes would be my armor at my new school, where I would finally be just another Asian girl among hundreds, my peacoat spun-wool proof that I belonged.

———

My mother used to proclaim loudly and often that there was nothing she missed about Ohio. Despite his pride in "getting out," I know there were things about it that my father felt nostalgic for, like attending the Region 4 Boy Scout camp every summer with his dad and brother, or cheering on Cleveland's sports teams with people who cared about them as much as he did. Our family couldn't afford to travel, and many of our relatives, especially those in Ohio, thought of Oregon as another planet, so I grew up knowing them as voices on the other end of a phone passed around at holidays. A born-and-bred New Englander once told me that if you picked up the country and shook it, people without deep roots anywhere else would fall to the West Coast. But my parents' roots in Cleveland ran deep, and even as a child I understood how easy it would have been for them to stay and build a life their families would have understood, surrounded by all that was familiar.

Instead, the earliest choices they made together took them far from home, a move they never regretted—they leaped without hesitation, much as they did when they decided to become parents through adoption, though they had little guidance from the child welfare system and no model for how to raise a Korean child as white parents. Perhaps it's no surprise that when they let me go, it was not with the grudging wonder of my father's family when they left Ohio, nor the secret shame of the birth parents who gave me up as a baby—they encouraged me because their priority was my happiness, even if the pursuit of it took me away from them. That they frequently saw promise where others might have seen only risk is something I cannot help but admire. Sometimes I wonder if being their child, a product of their choices and their faith if not their genes, is what made me believe that another life might be within my reach.

I also wonder if I would have felt the same need to uproot myself had I been one more white girl with good grades, my presence secure and unquestioned in the place I'd been planted. It would be simpler, less discomfiting, to embrace the notion that luck and drive, the desire to get an education and help my family, were the only factors in my flight; I would prefer not to give my racial isolation as an adoptee, or my early experiences with bigotry and bullying, any more weight. But I was a Korean girl, the only Korean girl I knew, growing up in a place where no one seemed to know quite what to make of me, and where others were quick to let me know that I was not wanted. I understood that I would leave long before I knew how I would manage it.

The day I left home as a sheltered, untested eighteen-year-old was far and away the most terrifying I'd ever known. It sits alongside my adoption as one of the most important crossroads in my life—the launching point for yet another attempted assimilation, although I didn't think of it that way at the time. Remembering that my parents had also made the decision to leave everything and everyone they knew behind, simply because they longed for a different kind of life and believed they would find it together, helped give me the courage I needed. To this day it remains one of their legacies to me, a strand connecting the very different lives we have led, reminding me that I am their child.

3

THINGS MY MOTHER SENT ME AFTER I LEFT HOME

Oregon postcards

Calling cards

Cash, when she had any to spare

Vitamins

Ballpoint pens and mechanical pencils

Post-it notes

Lip balm

Sunscreen

My favorite Girl Scout cookies

Enough Werther's Originals, Brach's peppermints,
and saltwater taffy for everyone in my dorm to help

themselves from my free-for-all candy dish, plus seasonal candy for holidays

A two-foot artificial Christmas tree, with decorations

Warm socks

Knit gloves

Wool scarves (she was very concerned that I was too soft for East Coast winters)

A manicure kit

DVDs of my two favorite movies, *Singin' in the Rain* and *Casablanca*

Seashells and sand dollars

Articles of potential interest snipped from the local newspaper

A flashlight

A safety whistle

Pepper spray

Photos of her and Dad and Grandma on every birthday and holiday I missed

4

"I'M GLAD THAT'S OVER."

Dan looked a little green as we made our way down the boarding stairs and across the tarmac to the airport entrance, backpacks slung over our shoulders. Our connecting flight from Portland had been bumpy, the plane cabin so small that we were unable to sit side by side; our seats were on opposite sides of an aisle so narrow the flight attendant couldn't squeeze a cart through. I was accustomed to such flights after four years of coast-to-coast travel—sometimes it was only me, one or two other passengers, the pilot, and a single attendant on the final leg of the trip down from PDX or up from SFO—but my husband, who had grown up near Hartford, apparently had little experience with puddle jumpers.

As usual on a day with no fog, I'd been able to spot the rooftops of my old neighborhood, if not my parents' exact roof, from the window of the plane. The house was in the direct path of nearly every flight that landed at our tiny regional airport, and my father liked to tell people that a few low fliers had clipped branches off the tallest trees in our backyard. I don't know if that was true—every third thing Dad said was intended as a joke, delivered so straight-faced that sometimes you couldn't tell—but I was used to hearing the roar of flight after flight overhead, descending planes shaking the windows of my childhood bedroom.

Growing up, I'd hardly ever invited anyone over to that house. My friends and I tended to rotate between homes that were larger and tidier than mine, where there was usually a parent around and where it was understood that our presence, our volume, and our ability to clear a pantry of snacks in minutes wouldn't be a burden. Even my grandmother, who lived twenty minutes away, did not come over unless she was picking me up; on holidays, we gathered at her house. It felt strange to be bringing a husband home to a place that had always been for my parents and me alone.

"Remember," I told him, "you're not allowed to divorce me based on anything that happens on this trip."

"I'm sure it's going to be great." Dan squeezed my hand as we walked through the gate, both of us already on the lookout for my family.

At twenty-two and twenty-three, we looked like college kids returning home, though it was the wrong time of year for that. We had married the previous summer, having not so much overcome as outlasted his parents' objections over how young we were. This was his first trip to Oregon, and I was very aware that we were doing things in the wrong, or at least unexpected, order. Shouldn't he have been home with me before now? But unlike his home, mine was so far away, and so hard to get back to, even when I wanted to go.

My parents were waiting for us on the other side of the security doors. "You made it!" Mom said, as she always did when I landed. She meant *you made it through your flights*, and also *you made it through however long it's been since your last visit*. She looked much the same as she had the last time I'd seen her, though her hair, once copper-red, now reddish-brown, was growing out from the pixie cut she'd had at my wedding. It was my father that I surveyed with an anxiety I tried not to let on. His dark hair had gone gray years ago, like that of all the men in his family, and his blue eyes were alight with happiness as my parents tackled us with hugs, but did he look more careworn than he had the last time we'd seen him? Before this trip, Mom told me that he'd been experiencing some health problems, "complications" from his diabetes—I thought she had mentioned his thyroid, too—but at first glance he seemed all right, steady on his feet as we moved toward the airport's only baggage carousel.

Anyone looking at our group might have assumed that Dan was my parents' child. Not that he looked much like either of them with his mother's thick dark hair and easy grin, though at a hair under six feet, he was exactly my dad's height—it was just that I looked nothing like any of them. I made my habitual survey of the room as we waited for our suitcases. As I'd expected, I was the only Asian in sight.

——

"The Jesuit missionaries didn't only see themselves as bringing the Catholic faith to Indigenous people, but 'civilizing' them. What does that really mean, to 'civilize' someone?" our professor asked, looking around the seminar table.

After a pause, I said, "To make them more like you."

I was the only freshman in a roomful of upperclassmen, and still found the rapid-fire discussion somewhat intimidating; my papers were well written, the professor had told me, but I should learn to speak up more often in class. Now he nodded at me, and I thought I read a trace of approval in the half smile accompanying his "yes."

In another class, the professor asked each of us to share where we were from. When I told her, assuming that the history of my home state would be largely irrelevant to our discussion of Jim Crow laws, she exclaimed, "Oregon! Speaking of racism," and launched into a mini-lecture on the state's founding as a racist white utopia. "Haven't you ever wondered why Oregon is so white?" she asked.

I had not. I loved history, even before I decided to major in it; I'd paid attention during social studies lessons and school field trips, and watched history documentaries for fun. In my thirteen years attending Oregon schools, I had learned about cultural genocide and the forceful displacement of the region's Indigenous communities and even heard whispers about nearby white supremacist groups, but had never been told that Black people were long forbidden to settle in Oregon, or that the state had levied a special tax on people of color, or that the legislature hadn't formally ratified the Fifteenth Amendment until 1959. As my professor spoke, I realized it was no unfortunate accident that I had grown up in such a homogeneous place; its prevailing whiteness was by design, a legacy of violent and exclusionary laws that functioned precisely as their architects had intended.

I doubt my parents were surprised when I came home and did what humanities students do so well: argue with anyone who will listen. We debated everything from American imperialism and nuclear proliferation to immigration and affirmative action, and they seemed to find some of my emerging views more amusing than troubling, although I do remember them informing me, more than once, that I had been "brainwashed" in college. They had been raised by blue-collar FDR Democrats, and my mother told me that she'd voted that way until Carter. By the time I was old enough to pay attention, both she and my father were independent voters who leaned libertarian—a result, perhaps, of living in a corner of the state that could feel stagnant and forgotten as its once-booming timber industry began to decline. Like many others we knew, my parents were highly critical of both the federal and state governments, and often said that no politician of any party could be trusted.

I suspect it came as a greater surprise to them when I began talking about racism within the context of my experience as a Korean American adoptee. This was personal to our family, and to them it might have appeared to come out of nowhere, though from my perspective I was only finding new language for things I'd witnessed and felt all my life. My parents would try, in later years, to accept what I told them about my experiences, but this was harder for all of us to speak about when I was nineteen. If they wanted to, they could maintain that race was largely inconsequential in people's daily lives. They could believe that there were few racists in our town because they had never been among their targets. They could ask me if I thought it was right or fair that so many immigrants were moving here, as if I were not the first person in my Korean family born on American soil.

My family had been instructed to take a "color-blind" approach to parenting. "Assimilate her into your family," the judge who finalized my adoption had told them—*make her more like you*—"and everything will be fine." They heard similar advice from their attorney and social workers. Throughout my childhood, I often struggled to understand myself as Korean in part because my white family, encouraged by such "experts," did not see my race or theirs as relevant within our household or outside it. I cannot recall a single conversation we had about anti-Asian prejudice, specifically—not the model-minority myth, not perpetual-foreigner syndrome, not the exotification and fetishization of Asian women, not the legacy of America's imperialist wars that was partially responsible for my birth family's and my presence here. The closest we came to talking about race when I was a child was my parents' assertion that they would have adopted me whether I was *Black, white, or purple with polka dots*. As a child, I was too confused and ashamed to tell them about the ongoing racism I experienced: the slurs and taunts from kids, the prying and thoughtless comments from adults. I was trying to protect both them and myself. I didn't know how to explain to them that the color blindness they claimed to espouse did not reflect reality as I knew it; that our experiences and views differed in part because I was Asian and they were not. I could no more make them understand how it felt to be a Korean American adoptee than they could transfer their whiteness to me.

There was another change, more sudden and less subtle, in my life as an adoptee after I left home: I never had to disclose my adoption to others unless I felt like it. When I did share it, people were sometimes curious, but the invasive questions, that objectifying fascination I'd encountered growing up, did not always follow. It was possible to lower some of the defenses I'd unknowingly built for my own protection as I began to reconsider the adoption story I'd been told since early childhood, wondering about the true impact of losing my roots and growing up in near-total racial isolation. It was still not a line of inquiry I found uncomplicated or comfortable. But it was one that I could finally begin to pursue once I'd left home, because I thought that it could not deeply wound my parents, nor threaten the stability of the adoptive family I felt such a strong obligation to defend, when I was no longer a child under their roof.

———

Dan stared out the window during the short drive to my parents' house, his expression one of wonder. I tried to view the land I'd known all my life through new eyes, his eyes. The Cascades and Siskiyous rose around us, every road lined in evergreens and deciduous trees in full late-summer leaf. My mother had turned off the lukewarm air-conditioning in her fifteen-year-old Nissan sedan and rolled the windows halfway down, and the cool September air was both a shock and a balm after the oppressive mid-Atlantic humidity we had left behind. We would need the sweatshirts and long pants we'd brought with us.

All I could remember about my last visit to Oregon was sitting at my parents' white Formica dining table, feeling helpless as I listened to my mother cry about my wedding.

My family supported our decision to marry, but Mom was upset that I wasn't getting married "from home." I was utterly blindsided by her disappointment—hosting was not something I thought my parents cared about. It wasn't that our family did not socialize, but we generally did not entertain. And why would I expect my parents to plan and host a wedding *here* when I lived three thousand miles away?

I tried to list all my logical reasons for marrying in our college town instead, the challenges of planning a wedding from across the country: Flights into our little airport would take forever and cost everyone outside Oregon—97 percent of our guests—a small fortune. I couldn't think of a local hotel to recommend. I couldn't visit venues or bakeries or florists here. I had no interest in getting married at the church I'd grown up attending; nor did I want to marry in the Orthodox parish my parents now belonged to, even if that would have been permitted. I did not tell my mother what I was really thinking, which was that by then I would have gladly canceled the wedding and eloped if I could have done so without breaking her heart.

You're ashamed, she said, skimming over every reason I'd given and going for the direct cut. *You don't want everyone to see where you grew up.* It was the first and only time I ever heard her say, *We're just your white-trash family.*

I was young, but I did know myself a little. And it was true that I had no desire to invite everyone I knew to whatever sort of function I might have been able to assemble, from a distance, in our town. I *was* conscious of the differences between Dan's family and mine, eager to win his parents' approval, and hoping to protect my own from judgment. But *ashamed, white trash*—these were words I had never used and didn't identify with. I couldn't understand why my mother had seized on them, why she would wield them like weapons against both of us.

None of my practical arguments moved her. She had always imagined me getting married at home, though she had never said so before, and now, for the first time in my life, I had let her down. I was sorry for it, though the hurt had been unintentional. But I was not remotely tempted to give in and move the wedding. My mother had not raised me to fear her disapproval or rejection; even as we argued, I understood that she loved me far too much to be unhappy at my wedding. What I couldn't seem to adequately express to her was that, practicality aside, it made no sense to me to celebrate one of the most important days of my life in a place to which I felt no strong connection. If my family hadn't lived there, I don't know that I ever would have gone back.

———

Growing up, I knew kids whose families belonged to the country club, kids who got new cars on their sixteenth birthdays, kids whose parents took them skiing every winter in Bend or Lake Tahoe. When I went to their houses, I would try out their expensive gaming systems and swim in their inground pools, notice their "nice" living rooms that, unlike their more casual "family rooms," were rarely used. Most of the time, it was easy to forget that most of my friends were from families with more money than mine, because I'd known them for years and because many rich people in Oregon dressed and acted exactly like the rest of us.

In college, markers of class had seemed starker and more numerous, from my friends' Armani Exchange shopping sprees to the multiple work-study jobs I held. I learned not to mention my scholarships to most people, not because I was embarrassed, but because I tired of hearing them say *you're so lucky!* while bemoaning the full tuition their parents "had" to pay. I participated in a dorm holiday gift swap one year and nearly panicked when I heard about the fifty-dollar suggested spending amount; not only was it more than I'd ever spent on a single gift for anyone, it was more than I had in my checking account. When we went out to an expensive restaurant to exchange our gifts, I ordered the cheapest thing on the menu and stuck to water, praying that no one would insist on splitting the bill.

Once I started working in the undergraduate admissions office, I was able to meet both the admissions officer who'd accepted me and the financial aid adviser who made my attendance possible. It was strangely reassuring to realize that they were not crusading do-gooders, merely academic administrators doing their jobs. I began to understand that it was in the school's best interest to accept promising students and try to make it possible for them to attend—which meant that I was not a charity case, even if I was also not the financial boon to the university that some were. When an admissions officer told a group of student volunteers, *You guys are all just tuition with feet, as far as I'm concerned*, I knew he was joking, though I did not laugh. I never forgot about my lack of money—even if I could have, regularly emptying my bank account to pay for books or make rent would have reminded me—but it rarely seemed important when I had friends, classes I loved, a place to live, and a meal plan.

I threw myself into every project and paper, joined clubs and gave campus tours, became a research assistant to one of my professors. Suddenly there seemed to be so little daylight between what I had and what I wanted, who I was and what I was doing—I wasn't one person in class and another in my private moments; for the first time, every part of my life felt integrated with the rest. I found myself considering a career in academia, something I don't think I could have done had I felt like a total impostor. Consumed with my studies and my social life, my world expanding beyond anything I'd been able to imagine, I rarely stopped to think about what it meant that I was now far more comfortable in the rarefied air of campus than I had ever been in my hometown.

Then I would fly back home and it would hit me anew, that cold prickle of awareness somewhere between my shoulder blades. I felt small and somehow trapped whenever I returned, as though I wouldn't be allowed to leave, even though I was only a visitor now, the interloper I'd always looked like. My visits got shorter and shorter, and it was impossible to ignore the mingled guilt and relief I felt every time I boarded a flight headed east. Campus was where I had a life, a purpose, new ideas to absorb—where things were always changing, where no one stared at me when I entered a room, where I no longer questioned the fact that I belonged.

———

We pulled up to my parents' house, a little white 1970s ranch house with rust-red shutters sitting at a bend in the road, where they had lived since the year before I was born. To the left, slanting high above the part of our yard my family called "the back forty," the rounded summit of one of the lesser but nearer peaks in the western Cascades loomed dark blue in the gathering dusk, appearing so close that I used to imagine we could walk right up to it from our house. Again, Dan admired the view, but I was focused on silently fretting as we followed my parents up the driveway. I was "home," and I wasn't; now, when I thought of *home*, I thought about the seven-hundred-square-foot city apartment where Dan and I lived.

Though he had never been to Oregon with me before, I'd now spent several holidays at his parents' home in Connecticut, which was far easier for us to reach. To me, one of seventeen guests they hosted one Thanksgiving, the trappings of their upper-middle-class life looked like wealth, although Dan had once jokingly referred to them as "your basic hardworking, flinty New Englanders"—by which he seemed to mean that while they didn't have to worry about money the way my family did, they kept the thermostat low in the winter, refused to get cable, and felt the impact of the sizable tuition checks they were able to write. Even when he and I were in the college bubble, leading lives that looked similar on the surface, I was aware that our experiences diverged in any number of ways. His parents probably outearned mine ten times over. He worked a campus job for extra cash, as I did, but if his bank account was getting low, funds were a phone call away. His number of trips home wasn't limited by the cost of plane tickets. He was meeting the status quo by going to a good university; he had multiple relatives with advanced degrees, familial expectations that went well beyond college. There was a reason that he was now applying to full-time graduate programs while I wavered, worried about subsisting on an academic stipend; we'd gone to the same school, had similar GPAs and former professors urging us toward further study, but our respective backgrounds led us to evaluate risks and opportunities quite differently.

Standing with him in my parents' living room, I took a moment to inventory both the familiar and the new: a different sofa, the same faded pale-pink carpet and off-white linoleum, different wallpaper, same popcorn ceiling. A few framed photos from our wedding had recently joined the many-years-old family portraits and knickknacks on the mantel. The furniture was in a new arrangement—my mother was never content with one for long—and there were no ashtrays anywhere; I recalled Mom telling me that she now made Dad take his cigarettes out on the cement patio. Fewer than a dozen steps brought us to the door of my old bedroom, which had undergone a complete transformation since my last visit, its walls painted white, its closet emptied, most of my books donated, stored elsewhere, or absorbed into my parents' collection. The need to make space for me and my new husband was evidently what had pushed them to clear out my old belongings. They had also acquired a queen-sized mattress, so we wouldn't have to squeeze into my old twin bed. It took up nearly all the floor space, leaving just enough room for a small bureau and a single nightstand.

The room was no longer my childhood bedroom but a generic guest room, the oval "tot finder" fire rescue sticker on the window the only evidence that a child had occupied it. My mom had once told me the sticker was there so the firefighters would know to save me first. I think she meant to reassure me, but I remember worrying that I would be saved and my parents wouldn't be. Now I opened the window to wedge my old box fan in place, turning it to the highest setting, enveloping the room in white noise.

Later that night, I woke from sleep to a loud gasp beside me. I turned to see what had startled Dan, and then began to laugh: Sebastian, my fluffy gray cat, was sitting squarely on his chest. I'd gotten Sebastian as a pitiful runty, dirty kitten when I was nine years old, and he'd been my joy and treasure, sleeping with me for part of the night before he got up to prowl. He wasn't too proud to come when I called him at the back door, even after months away; when I visited, he would take up his old post in my room, though my parents said he ignored it when I was at school. Now a cat of advanced years, he peered down at my husband with what I imagined was a crotchety but curious mien: *I know who she is, I remember her. Now who the hell are you?* Dan, who would take much in stride that week, laughed and gave Sebastian's ears a scratch, and my old cat immediately began to purr.

———

The day after meeting Dan, my parents had taken me to a furniture store near campus. Now a junior, I had recently moved out of the dorm and into a small apartment in a hundred-year-old building, and the only furniture I had was a twin bed and a cheap white laminate desk. As we walked through the aisles, looking at shelves and dressers, my mother said, "I think Dan has decided that he's going to marry you."

"Stop," I told her.

"You always used to say that you'd only marry someone

smarter than you." Her voice had taken on the gleeful pitch it did whenever she was teasing me, or reminding me of what an absolute dork I'd been. I couldn't remember saying that to her, but now it struck me as insufferable: What had I even meant by it? How had I imagined that I would judge such a thing? Why were we talking about marriage at all?

"We're smart in different ways," I said feebly, which made her laugh.

In truth, I thought Dan was probably smarter than me, though he was so good-natured—funny, quick to smile or let out a laugh louder than his natural speaking voice, kind and approachable in his glasses and rotating selection of T-shirts—that in the early weeks of our friendship I nearly overlooked how brilliant he was. He had a strong competitive streak, I soon learned—in classes filled with future doctors and engineers, he liked setting the curve; when we played games, he always wanted to win—but he was also far more interested in what he didn't know than what he did, patient and unfailingly steady. What made me start to think that his was perhaps not the same run-of-the-mill intelligence nearly everyone we knew in college possessed was watching him explain an organic chemistry lesson to a group of friends. He was a natural teacher, able to break things down step-by-step in a way I was sure I'd never been able to do with any mate-rial, even material I knew quite well, but what impressed me most was how readily he offered assistance to anyone who needed help, without expecting anything in return.

I have the better memory by far, but to this day he can tell you what I was wearing when we met. We found that we had the same odd lunch break, an hour later than most people we knew, so it seemed only natural to meet up for lunch. Soon we were hanging out several evenings a week, doing homework together despite having none of the same classes. He was quieter than I was, but we never ran out of conversation; I always had another question, another story, something he seemed to enjoy. It feels significant that I met him at a time when I felt perfectly satisfied with my little life on campus, sufficient unto myself. I figured I wasn't missing out on anything by not seriously dating in college, particularly after watching some friends go through breakups that threatened to derail their whole semester; I was happier than I had ever been, and every day felt like an affirmation of my decision to let my classes and my friendships be what sustained me. I soon realized that being with Dan, whether we were talking or working in silence, was as effortless as being alone, if considerably more fun. I felt more like myself in his company, which was of course partly why I had been seeking it out so often.

Still, I was surprised when a mutual friend told me that he had feelings for me. No, we were just good friends, I insisted—friends who hung out several days a week, who, okay, had maybe held hands once or twice, but in a totally friendly, casual way? "Dating would ruin our friendship," I said. "I'm happy, I'm busy, and I don't need any drama."

"Okay," she said. "So you'd be fine with him dating someone else then."

Like who? What had she heard?

My mother laughed loud and long when I told her that we were "serious" after a month or so of dating, probably because I'd spent the entire year before insisting that college was no time to be looking for commitment. It did feel early for him to meet my parents when they flew out from Oregon a month later, but it was the one and only time they had managed to visit me on campus, and I had no idea when I'd have another chance to introduce him. The four of us went out to dinner, and the next day we all worked on putting my new dresser and bookshelves together. Watching him with my parents, I found myself thinking that the immediate ease he'd established with them had to be a good sign—also the fact that he had watched us interact and tease and annoy each other for two days, and none of it appeared to scare him off.

I recalled a day in tenth grade when some friends and I had taken turns making predictions for each other, trying to imagine our lives after high school. Maria was going to be a marine biologist, Kristie was going to be a teacher or a park ranger, I'd be a journalist, and we'd have a couple of kids each. *You'll definitely be the last of us to get married,* another friend told me, *if you get married at all.* She thought my standards would be *too high* and I'd probably be focused on my career. I remember laughing, wondering if I was being complimented, feeling warm because my friends and I knew each other well enough to dream on one another's behalf. But even then, I'd told them that I hoped to have a partner and children someday. The possibility of creating a different kind of family, one I would not have to question my place in, had long been appealing to me as an adoptee, and I knew that I might never have the experience of seeing a face like mine unless I had a child of my own.

Though my parents were traditionalists at heart, they were not the sort to pressure me into a certain kind of life.

My mother told me that she didn't care when or whether I got married. *Just remember,* she would always say, *you're not allowed to get married without me there.*

I'm sure my parents wouldn't have hesitated to tell me if they had reservations about Dan. They liked him instantly, but more than that, they trusted him; after that first meeting, they would consider him part of the family, treating him like a son before it was official. Now I can only guess at the reasons behind their instinctive acceptance of him, their unwavering faith in our relationship. I'm sure they saw how much he loved and respected me. That I felt certain of him—so certain that I would bet my future on us, never seeing our decision to marry as the risk it undoubtedly was—was something I imagine they must have understood at least in part because of the life they chose when they married and left home. They weren't used to seeing me so content; they would have remembered how hard I'd pushed myself as a teenager, the fact that I was never satisfied with anything I did. I believe they were both surprised and pleased to discover I was open to a kind of happiness that didn't entirely hinge on where I might flee to or what I might achieve.

You've always known what was right for you, my mother said.

I have wondered if I should feel embarrassed for marrying so young. I've never been able to muster up any regret. Not long ago, I mentioned to Dan that I think I have been at least four or five different people in the years he's known me, and after giving it a little thought, he was able to name every iteration I was thinking of, every distinct stage and transformation of the last two decades. If there is a constant in my adult life, it is that he has always seen me, respected me, and loved me completely. We knew so little of ourselves or the world when we got married, but we were right to believe that we could change and grow together and make each other happy.

I have no doubt that my parents would have relished having more time as my primary family, the people I thought of as *home*. They could have chosen to disapprove of or resent me when I made choices that they did not anticipate, choices that kept me far away from them. But their love for me was never about ownership, or control, or whether I followed the path they expected. They were grateful that Dan and I had found each other, and they weren't afraid that we would struggle, because they themselves had not experienced a life free from struggle. *We're lucky*, my father said in his wedding toast, *to get to witness your love and commitment. We can't wait to see the life you'll build together.* They never saw me as choosing one kind of family over another, one dream or one life over another. They could not imagine a future in which I did not pursue everything I wanted.

We drove all over the region with my parents that week, taking advantage of the good weather and the timing of our trip; mountain roads that would have been impassable during the winter months were clear and open in early fall, and the occasional drizzle didn't deter us. Mom made us pose for pictures in front of a lighthouse, at the seaside botanical gardens she loved, on a bridge stretching over a rushing river gorge. My anxiety eased as the visit wore on, and it was a pleasant surprise to discover how much I enjoyed reacquainting myself with our little corner of the Northwest; time and distance had increased my appreciation, and I forgot to feel trapped or out of place when I saw my husband wide-eyed at the deep cerulean beauty of Crater Lake, the serene glory of a redwood grove, the wild cliffs overlooking the Pacific. I took pleasure in being the one to introduce him to these places I felt an uncomplicated love for, places that had been a familiar solace to me growing up.

Sometimes, though, I noticed that my father would lag a bit behind or wait in the car while the rest of us tackled a trail. There were nights when he would pick small, petty fights with me, the way he sometimes did when his blood sugar was uncontrolled and his mood fluctuated as a result. Hurt, confused, I argued back, simultaneously angry and embarrassed that Dan was there to witness our bickering. In calmer moments, when I asked Dad if he was feeling all right, the most he'd admit to was being *a little tired*.

Mom quietly told me that he was experiencing some neuropathy in his feet. His eyesight was worsening, too; he needed a new prescription. I don't remember if I thought to ask whether he was getting the treatment and medications he needed. I know I watched him more closely after that, but he didn't seem to have any trouble maneuvering around the house or the neighborhood.

It was the last time I would return to my childhood home, although I didn't know it then. Soon my parents would sell the house and move into a manufactured home fifteen minutes up the highway, with a view of different mountains. By the time our visit with them was over, I felt foolish for having worried about it. My family had been overjoyed to see us, and Dan, easygoing middle child that he was, had not been remotely fazed by our little squabbles. I could almost imagine bringing our future kids back here one day, showing them the sights. Sometimes, looking at my mother, I felt sure that she was picturing the same.

5

MY FATHER HAD TRIED HIS FIRST CIGARETTE ON A DARE
from an older kid when he was thirteen, he told me one day,
and had never given it up. I remember the conversation because he spoke so seriously, with none of his usual humor,
almost as if he were giving a speech. He looked embarrassed
when he told me about accepting the dare because the other
kid called him a chicken, though he recovered enough to
tell me that if he ever caught me smoking, I'd be sorry. We
had learned about the dangers of smoking in elementary
school, and I had nightmares about my father's lungs filling
with tumors, him struggling to breathe. For a few determined weeks when I was eight or nine, I tried leaving notes
around the house that read *SMOKING CAUSES CAN-
CER*, an idea I'd stolen from a Ramona book. "Everyone
in his family smokes, and none of them have gotten lung
cancer," Mom finally said one day, in an attempt to get me to
stop worrying, and also to stop throwing away Dad's cigarettes, because it made him apoplectic and of course never

stopped him from buying more. "That's not what people die of in his family."

I knew of my two absent grandparents, my dad's mom and my mom's dad, only from stories told by family members; both had died when I was a baby. My maternal grandfather's cancer spread fast, killing him in months. But while I remembered being told that my paternal grandmother was sick for most of my father's life, her pain dragged out across decades, I couldn't remember hearing why she died. I felt a jolt of morbid curiosity. "What do they die of, then?"

"It's their kidneys," Mom said. "And the diabetes."

She was correct about my father's genetic inheritance; by the time he was in his early forties, he and two of his siblings would be diagnosed with diabetes. I read the pamphlets Dad brought home from the doctor, extracting promises from him about how he would learn to manage the disease. But there was much that proved beyond his power to control. The medication he'd been prescribed was expensive without insurance and also upset his stomach, so he stopped taking it, saying that he couldn't work and serve food all day while feeling nauseated. As restaurant manager, he was usually the last one who got to take a break or eat lunch, and when he did get a meal, the food most readily available were the pizzas he helped make. He had little free time for regular exercise, no extra money to give to a gym or a nutritionist, and unless he felt very ill, he did not go to the doctor.

During the long years when he could trace no significant or debilitating issues to his condition, I doubt he had either the luxury or the inclination to worry much about his health—or his lack of health care. Even when both my parents found themselves unemployed in their late fifties, their initial worry was not for Dad's missed checkups but whether they would be able to pay their bills, cover their rent, buy groceries and gas. That is, until my father grew very sick, the sickest he had ever been, and we had no way of figuring out what was wrong with him.

———

We had been living in North Carolina for five years and Dan was close to finishing his dissertation when I gave birth to our second child. With her dark brown eyes, full-moon cheeks, and impressive rolls, she looked so much like her older sister that everyone in the family would mix up their baby pictures for years. We found the transition from one to two kids challenging, though in infancy our younger child seemed easier and less particular than our first had been, content to be curled up sleeping on one of us or carted around the house as we played with our busy three-year-old, who gabbed to her little sister as if hoping for a response. I bargained with God over the kids' opposing sleep schedules; Dan went from one cup of coffee per day to two. But we knew how to take care of a baby this time, and we also knew that newborn days were fleeting, and we'd miss them when they were over.

My parents were supposed to arrive for a visit not long after the birth. A couple of days before their trip, Mom called to tell me that Dad wasn't feeling well enough to travel. I hadn't realized he was feeling that poorly, but when I questioned my parents, neither wanted to discuss his health at length. Mom would make the trip alone, she said, though she was anxious about leaving my father. She decided to shorten her visit from two weeks to one.

My father's last steady job had been at a cell carrier call center, where, extrovert that he was, well trained in customer service thanks to his years working in restaurants, he'd enjoyed the work and found it easier than many of his previous jobs. After the center closed, he had stocked warehouse shelves for a snack food company and worked at a different call center before that one, too, shut down. When nothing else came along, my parents' tiny nest egg—what had been left after they sold their house, dispensed with some debt, and bought their new home—began to dwindle.

The last time I'd seen Dad, I had noticed that he was beginning to shuffle more than stride. Since then, he had reportedly given up most of his physical activities—his gardening, the walks he used to take around the neighborhood. Though he was still looking for work and insisted that he did not want to apply for Social Security Disability Insurance, I didn't know if he could work a full-time job anymore. When she came out to visit us, Mom said she thought his decline must be related to his diabetes, but they couldn't know for sure what was wrong until he saw a specialist. She assured me he would get to it; they had only recently secured health coverage through her job after a long stretch without it and were still catching up on appointments.

Toward the end of her stay, she got a call from her boss. She had been laid off with no notice or severance pay. The company couldn't even wait until she returned from vacation to give her the news. "This way, at least, you're eligible for unemployment benefits right away," her boss said. My parents' health plan would expire in days.

———

Once, while home on break from college, I asked my father what it was like being an empty nester. He admitted that it was "weird" and he was still getting used to it. "You spend eighteen years focused on raising a kid," he said, "and then one day everything changes."

"Do you think it'll ever feel normal?" I asked.

He shrugged. "Maybe. If you move back home."

We could have tried to move out west once Dan finished his doctoral program. But my academic goals had given us our next coordinates, and they were no closer to Oregon. I had been admitted to a creative writing graduate program in Washington, D.C., deferring enrollment by a year to get us through the newborn period and Dan's dissertation defense. While the thought of going back to school with an infant and a toddler at home was daunting, I was afraid that my creativity and drive would atrophy beyond recovery if I didn't at least try. Dan found a postdoctoral fellowship in the D.C. area, and we rented a town house within walking distance of his job. He made sure to get home in time for me to catch the train to my evening classes.

My parents' situation was worsening, and we were unable to help. Every cent we made went to basic living expenses—rent was three times what our monthly mortgage payment had been in North Carolina, and now we had preschool tuition to pay. There were many months when we had to put a little on our credit card to get by. My parents refused to take any

money from us, knowing that we would feel the pinch ourselves.

By now, Dad had bad neuropathy in his hands and feet,
sleep apnea, vision and dental problems. Some days, Mom
said, he couldn't walk across the street without getting tired.
But then, she added, his blood sugar wasn't the highest it had
ever been, and she didn't think the diabetes could fully explain the recent swelling in his legs, his aches and pains, his
upset stomach, or his persistent exhaustion. "He's only sixty,
and he looks and moves like an old man," she told me.

Not knowing what else to do, we both pushed my father
to apply for Social Security Disability Insurance. It took the
better part of two years, his longest-ever stretch of unemployment, to convince him. He had worked all his life and still
thought he could, if the right job came along. He only agreed
to apply for disability benefits when he began feeling so fa-
tigued that he had to spend much of the day sleeping. I don't
think I imagined the quiet note of satisfaction in his voice
when he called and told me that his claim had been denied, on
the grounds that he was not disabled, only unemployed. He
wanted me to know that I'd been wrong to pressure him—he
had put his hand out, and it had all been for nothing.

———

As a relatively young parent—our second child was born the
year I turned thirty—I'd once imagined that my own kids
would be mostly raised by the time my parents needed significant support. With my father's health deteriorating for
reasons we could not discern, I struggled to accept how little
I could do for him and my mother, my attention and ener-

gies divided between the family I was raising and the one that raised me. My parents were among the forty-eight million Americans at the time with no health insurance, and Dad was clearly in desperate need of medical attention. I couldn't bear to hear the strangling worry in my mother's voice, the exhaustion in my father's. Was this how he had felt when his mother was dying in Ohio and he was on the other side of the country?

I tried to help them research available assistance, though I knew how they felt about government programs. They might as well have spared themselves the time and trouble of applying for all the good it did: They were denied Medicaid coverage under the Oregon Health Plan. They were still too young to qualify for Social Security and Medicare based on age. They were ineligible for food and rental assistance. If they'd had dependents, a higher cost of living, it would be different, one social worker told them, but as it was, well, they both just needed to find work.

"I heard that nearly everyone is denied disability benefits the first time," I said to my mother on the phone one evening. "You can appeal the decision. Maybe you should talk to a lawyer." I didn't even notice that I was saying *you* and not *you and Dad*, a subconscious acknowledgment of the fact that much of the work, if there was an appeal, would fall to her.

"Your father has refused. You know how much applying and then being turned down hurt his pride. He doesn't think he's disabled."

"But he *is*. And we both know he needs to see a doctor. What about taking him to a community health clinic?"

A few years before, in the same month I gave birth to my first child, I'd reconnected with my Korean family and forged a relationship with my sister, Cindy. The health clinic she worked at served many poor and uninsured patients in the Portland area. When I told her about my parents' situation, she had suggested that we try to find a similar clinic near them, one that would charge on a sliding scale or perhaps offer my father free care.

"I've heard awful things from friends about one of the clinics here," Mom said. "They could kill him as easily as help him."

To me, this sounded like an excuse. "It would be better than not having him seen at all! He's getting worse. You have to do *something*."

Even as I spoke, my voice climbing in frustration, I knew that I had no right to try to give her orders. But Dad was sick, and she wasn't, so she had to take charge now. Who else could do it?

"What do you expect me to do, Nicole?" Her voice broke, and I hated myself for what I heard in her tone. Not the anger, which I understood, but that pitch of helpless fear. "I'm dealing with *way* more than I can handle already," she told me. "I'm doing the best I can."

I knew that she was terrified, stretched beyond her limit. She was still looking for work, too, and had been selling her plasma, something I could not persuade her to stop doing because we both knew I had no way to replace that income. It was her use of the singular *I* as much as her choked anxiety that made my eyes fill. She *was* alone. I'd made sure of that. What right did I have to suggest anything to her?

My parents never accused me of negligence, or being a terrible daughter. Sometimes I almost wished they would, because what they did felt even worse: they never asked me for anything. They seemed to have no expectations of me at all. When I fretted, when I offered what little help I could, they always said they didn't want me to worry about them. *Stop*, Mom would tell me. *You have your own family to take care of.*

As a kid, I could not remember envying people who had more money than we did. If I wished for something others had, it was the way most white people I knew could go about their lives in our part of Oregon unnoticed. By high school, I was aware that my family did not seem to have quite *enough*—enough to pay off debt, or stop my parents from worrying, or keep every unforeseen problem from turning into an emergency. But I had been fortunate in so many ways, shielded from serious hardship, protected by my parents and by others. If I had known this was coming for my father, my mother—if I had understood that things likely wouldn't get better for them after I left, only worse, and Dad wouldn't be able to get the medical care he needed—would I have made different choices? Who, exactly, would have warned me, helped me plan and figure out what I had to do to take better care of them?

I felt my frustration and uselessness with every shaky breath. If I kept pushing, I knew that I would only make things harder for my mother. But there had to be some way I could help.

"What if I call the clinic and make an appointment for him?" I said at last. "That's easy for me to do from here. Whatever their fee is, I'll pay it."

I heard her sigh. "You don't have to do that," she told me. "I will find time this week to call the clinic and get us an appointment."

She woke Dad from a nap and put the phone on speaker so he could say hello, and though he was too tired to talk for long, it was good to hear his voice, each of us striving to sound cheerful for the other's sake. Relieved, I let my parents draw me into conversation about the kids. I had been so focused on getting my father to see a doctor, *any* doctor, that it was difficult for me to think beyond the promised appointment. Even after all I'd heard about how sick he was, I couldn't imagine that he might be facing anything like his mother's illness, one that would render him a permanent patient and change my parents' lives yet again. He needed help to better manage his diabetes, I thought, or maybe he needed a different medication. The community clinic was the first step; soon, we'd learn how to make him well again.

6

SEVERAL YEARS AGO, WHEN I KNEW I WAS ABOUT TO BE laid off from an indie website that was shuttering, I received a statement from Discover claiming that Dan and I owed them more than fourteen hundred dollars. Neither of us had ever had a Discover card. The first customer service representative I spoke with clearly didn't believe me when I told her this, though she did feel sorry for me.

"Is there any chance that you might have opened the account and forgotten about it?" she asked gently.

I assured her there was *no* chance of that. We were living as frugally as we could with two children, finally beginning to recover from our combined years of graduate school, but we had nothing to spare, and I was soon to be unemployed. The rational part of my brain knew the card wasn't ours, and neither were the charges, and we probably couldn't be forced to pay fourteen hundred dollars plus interest if we hadn't been the ones to spend it. Still, I had grown up hearing my parents' warnings about credit card debt, and now felt myself edging closer to panic: What if the unexplained charges kept coming and we had to pay all of them? What if we were victims of identity theft and couldn't prove it and our credit was ruined and we were never able to rent a house or buy a car again?

By the time Dan got home, I was talking to another Discover representative, my agitation mounting. It took two minutes for my husband to get the story from me, take the phone, and confirm that we had received the statement in error. The company had no idea why or how our information had been associated with the account, which did belong to someone, just not to us. They promised to send us something in writing verifying that we didn't owe them anything. *Sorry for the inconvenience. Have a great evening.*

Dan handed my phone back to me, greeted the kids, and started making dinner, as usual. I expect that he forgot about the bill by the next morning. For days, I watched the mail, looking for the promised written confirmation that our errant debt had been cleared.

——

I have never been at ease when I think about money. I can acknowledge the necessity of it, try to earn and save it, share it with others who need it, but having to talk about or seriously plan around it will always make me feel small and afraid. A friend once asked me how much I would need to have in the bank to no longer worry, and I could only laugh. *More than I'll ever have.*

No one in my family had ever gone to graduate school, and I did not fully anticipate what several years of not maximizing our income, facing every shock and setback without a practical safety net, would mean. When my company laid me off while I was on maternity leave, we found ourselves temporarily living on Dan's graduate stipend. We expected some relief once he graduated and found a postdoc, but because we'd moved to a far more expensive area and I'd gone back to school, things felt as tight as they had before. Even after I landed another editorial position with a small website and ramped up my freelancing, we couldn't afford full-time child care for two young children. I learned to juggle my job duties and classwork around my older daughter's preschool schedule and early intervention services for our younger daughter, who was diagnosed with developmental delays at age two, autism at three. Without the flexibility of remote work, I might not have been able to work at all.

As fortunate as I have been compared to many, my creative career path is a difficult one for me to recommend. Stable editorial and writing jobs can be scarce, and I spent many years in low-paying roles with nice titles, working long hours for independent publishers with limited budgets. At times, I think my background made me more reluctant to negotiate—I was earning more than my parents had ever made; shouldn't I just be grateful to have this dream of a job, working with fellow writers, helping them tell the stories that mattered most to them? Shouldn't I feel glad to be in the room at all, especially when so few people in that room looked like me?

It feels important to acknowledge that any financial strain my husband and I have experienced has been born of our own luck, choices we were privileged to make. Our "broke" bore no resemblance to my parents' "broke," because ours was finite and because we always had other options: we could have quit our graduate programs, avoided having children, tried to pursue more lucrative careers. But when you have no savings and your debt is increasing, your anxious brain doesn't care that you chose the situation. Each month that we were a little short of what we needed, each year that I couldn't afford to fly my parents out to see us or go see them in turn, I felt a terrible, squeezing guilt—not only because I was failing them, but because I had yet to make the most of all the opportunities I'd been given.

We're often told that we will rise, reap the rewards, if only we work hard, have faith, wait our turn. What I wish I'd understood sooner is that my family didn't have time to wait. I will always be thankful that a substantial raise and my first book royalty check finally allowed me to help my mother. It all came too late to be of any use to my father.

———

I am still anxious when making a big purchase, whether it is necessary or not, and usually have to work myself up to justifying it. *The car is fifteen years old, the air conditioner can't be repaired, it's too small for all of us to be comfortable on long road trips → expenditure reluctantly approved*. I tend to choose smaller, less important things—sneakers, nightstands, the number of streaming services we pay for—to be stingy about, as if that will compensate for money I'm forced to spend elsewhere. If I want to splurge on something, I will tell myself that I have to take on a freelance assignment or speaking engagement, earn additional income, to make up for it. And yet I feel an undeniable thrill when I buy "nice things" for myself or for others, because to me it will always seem like a luxury to spend money on something I want but don't strictly need.

In contrast, my husband's approach to finances is rational, evenhanded, devoid of fear or strong emotion. He's never had a meltdown over math. He can see the numbers in the columns for what they are: incoming funds, outgoing expenses, things we want, and things we need. He does not find himself worrying or becoming upset because our kids, like many, do not yet understand the advantages they have. Even when we discuss how much money we might need to be able to retire someday—or potentially provide for our disabled child after we're dead—he doesn't panic. While both his family and mine might have described themselves as "middle class," there's an ocean, deep and wide, between our formative experiences around money and stability, and this disparity continues to influence our instincts and decisions around saving and spending.

I know it's a good thing that he doesn't make financial decisions from the same bottomless well of worry I do, but sometimes I can't help but envy his sense of security, the reassurance that comes with a lifetime of believing that you will most likely be okay. Witnessing his calm consistency can also make me feel foolish for fretting, though he would never condemn me for it. I tell myself that I should be able to recognize how lucky I am, put away these fears once and for all. I remind myself that I *have* taken risks, made decisions that were neither frugal nor practical, and it wasn't the end of the world: my financial anxiety couldn't override my desire to become a parent, a notoriously expensive proposition; nor did it stop me from pursuing a career in writing, a job that supports me now but might not a year from now. I did these things despite assuming, for years, that I might also need to be my parents' retirement plan.

Yet even when things are going well, I half expect to lose what I have. Some people claim this is because I am a "pessimist" while my husband is an "optimist," a framework that would seem to reduce my anxiety around money to an unfortunate personality quirk—if only I could relax, I'd be so much happier! In reality, there's a reason that he worries far less than I do, opens bills without dread, generally believes that things will work out in the end: he is from a family for whom things *do* work out. There's also a reason why he is unlikely to find himself staring up at the ceiling at two in the morning, interrogating every decision he's ever made: his family never needed something he couldn't provide because of the choices we made. Mine did.

While we spent a decade taking turns in graduate school, starting a family, pursuing what we believed were our dream careers, my father's health continued to decline. Never mind helping my parents when they needed it most; I could barely afford to visit them. They saw us once a year at most, sometimes every other year. They were the ones continually shortchanged—the parents we rarely saw, the grandparents who mostly watched their grandchildren grow up in photographs. It was devastating for them, and for me, and would have been even if those years had not turned out to be among my father's last.

7

THERE WERE TWO COMMUNITY HEALTH CLINICS WITH sliding pay scales within driving distance of my parents, both with long waiting lists. True or not, my mother had heard that one of them was dirty and understaffed, the providers negligent, so she called the other clinic and got my father an appointment. By calling when she did, she saved his life.

After giving my father a full examination and ordering blood work, the doctor got him an appointment with a kidney specialist who rotated through the clinic. The nephrologist was the one who finally diagnosed him with end-stage renal failure. "Your kidneys have lost over 90 percent of their function," he told my father. "You should have been on dialysis already. If you hadn't come in when you did, you'd be dead in weeks."

Even with a diagnosis and an order to begin dialysis, Dad had no health insurance to cover the ongoing treatments. "I'm going to connect you with a nurse at my office," the specialist said. "We're going to get you on disability and

Medicaid. They may have turned you down before, but they won't now." My parents were doubtful—they had reason to be—but within the week a nurse had helped my father submit another claim, and he was soon approved for Social Security Disability Insurance and the Oregon Health Plan. Though we knew the approval had only gone through because he was gravely ill, it still felt like something to celebrate.

His dialysis sessions would be outpatient, three days a week, at a nearby center. For his first treatment, he had to go to the hospital, where they would work up to the full four-hour session and watch him for any adverse reactions. When I called him at the hospital, he was watching *Monday Night Football* on the television in his room. He tried to reassure me—*It doesn't hurt at all, honey*—but he couldn't hide his anxiety. I knew how much he hated hospitals, and was at last beginning to understand how scarred he'd been by his mother's long illness and all the changes it wrought in his family. We chatted until he told me he was tired, and I hung up with my heart feeling bruised.

Slowly, with dialysis doing the work his kidneys could not, he began to feel a little better, a little stronger. Sometimes he took advantage of the free medical van service available to him, but often he was able to drive himself to the treatment center and back. Mom found part-time work again, doing light bookkeeping three days a week for a local counseling practice, and told me that her new employers were the nicest people she had ever worked for. Thanks to her steady paycheck and my father's improving health, they felt able to book flights out to see us.

Dad found the nearest dialysis center and continued his treatments during their stay. Each morning, before he left for the center, I would watch him pack a large-print novel, an audiobook, and a paper bag filled with snacks—carrot sticks, apple slices, cheese, and multigrain crackers—to get him through the hours hooked up to the dialysis machine. I noticed that he usually took a long nap after getting home. I worried every time he had to climb the seven or eight steps to the door of our rented town house; he took stairs in the same way our toddler did, a half step at a time. To me, he still looked and seemed older than his sixty-one years. But it was a relief to know that he was managing better; that he was no longer considered to be at death's door.

Now that my eldest was four, she could actually understand many of my father's quips. *I'm hungry*, she might say, and he would shake her hand and say, very seriously, *Hi, Hungry, nice to meet you*. Sometimes, when he was doling out jokes, she couldn't even speak through her laughter, and I smiled, thinking of how thrilled he must be that she found him so much funnier than I did. How had I forgotten how genuinely great my father was with kids? There was a reason he was the one asked to dress up as Saint Nicholas and hand out treats to children at my parents' parish at Christmastime.

A few weeks after my parents had returned home, I summoned the courage to look up *life expectancy on dialysis*, and learned that the average time I could expect him to live was five to ten years.

———

Like other patients with end-stage renal failure, including his mother before him, my father had to decide whether to continue with dialysis indefinitely or try to get a kidney transplant. If he chose a transplant, he could take his chances on the wait list and hope for a kidney from a recently deceased or altruistic donor—though he was warned that it was a long shot given the shortage of donor kidneys, and he would need to quit smoking to be eligible—or he could try to match with a family member.

He was entirely opposed to accepting a stranger's kidney. "I don't think I could live with it," he told my mother. "I'd always wonder if that meant some younger person, someone with kids still at home, didn't get one."

That left the option of a donation from a family member, but none of his siblings were healthy enough to donate. He wouldn't hear of my mother or me undergoing donor testing. I had kids to think about, he insisted, and his health wasn't worth the risk to mine. With typical impatience, I told him he shouldn't be so dramatic, none of us were going to die from giving him a kidney, but he refused to consider it.

"Dialysis isn't that bad," he said. "For now, I'll take my chances with it."

I may never know all the reasons why he didn't feel more open to receiving a donated kidney, whether from a family member or from a stranger. Though I've often wished that we could have come up with an argument that would have changed his mind, my mother believed nothing either of us could say would have swayed him. She said that he remembered his mother's agony after organ rejection, and in the end he believed that neither dialysis nor a transplant would give him a long life.

The dialysis did its job, as it had for his mother, first saving and then extending his life. But the ongoing treatments left him drained and far more vulnerable to other illnesses and infections. His immune system was compromised; he was constantly getting sick. We knew that he wasn't thriving, nor was he improving. He was enduring.

———

He had been on dialysis for four and a half years when he began experiencing balance problems, head and neck pain, difficulty walking. After two painful falls and a high fever, he finally made an appointment with his doctor. An MRI showed an aggressive case of osteomyelitis, a bone infection, in his vertebrae, which was putting pressure on his neck and attacking his spinal cord. The doctor wasn't certain where it had come from; while the area around his dialysis port was vulnerable to infection, it appeared to be clear. His best guess was that the bacterial attack might have started in the teeth and gums, where my father was prone to abscesses and infections. Both diabetes and dialysis increased his risk of dental problems, and he had rarely had access to comprehensive dental coverage.

My father was referred to a neurosurgeon, who performed surgery within hours. "If you wait even one more day, you're risking paralysis or spinal stroke," he told my parents. He removed a badly inflamed spinal disk and several damaged vertebrae, putting in plates and screws where necessary.

The operation was successful, but when Dad woke up in the recovery area, he kept clearing his throat, insisting he "could feel something down there." Soon his trachea was so swollen from the infection and the trauma of the operation that he needed to be intubated and moved to the ICU. All of this happened so quickly that my mother had no time to update me. By the time she could call, the swelling had gone down, and Dad was off the ventilator and breathing on his own again.

She agreed that we should try to come out and visit soon, but advised us to wait until he came home from the hospital. "There'd be nothing for you to do right now," she said, sounding impossibly weary. When I was able to talk to Dad, I spent most of the call in tears, apologizing for not being closer. It was still hard for him to speak. He tried to tell me that it was all right, he was getting the care he needed, and he knew that I was praying for him and doing what I could. But his voice broke as he said the words.

Two weeks later, in June, he was allowed to come home with a walker and a neck brace. We flew out to visit; Dan's parents helped with the cost of the short-notice trip. I could see how much ground my dad had lost, how much pain he was in. I tried to tell myself, as I often had before, that the worst was over and he would recover. Even after laying eyes on him, I did not understand how severely the infection had weakened him.

8

ONE WEEK INTO THE NEW YEAR, I WAKE TO SEE THAT I
missed two calls in the night. There is a voice mail from my
aunt, seven seconds long.

"Nicole, when you get this message, call your mom right
away. Your father died last night."

The absence of comprehension is its own kind of anguish.
I cannot say how I feel, or if I do. Later, I will understand
that this is no emotional void, but shock, sudden and over-
powering. A question pushes its way up through my numb,
grasping mind. *If Dad is dead*—No. He isn't—*why wasn't my
mother the one to call me?*

I get out of bed and stand shivering in my thin black
nightgown, phone gripped in my hand. Down the hall, I can
hear my children talking as they eat breakfast. I could call for
Dan, seek out his comfort before doing anything else. But
what will I tell him? What will I tell my kids when they ask
me what happened?

I call my parents' landline and my mother answers, her voice a splinter of itself—hoarse from crying, I assume. "Mom?" I say, my voice shaking, and she says, "Yes, it's me," as if I wouldn't recognize her. "I have laryngitis," she tells me.

I can't bring myself to ask how he died. I can't say the words *dead* or *died* at all. "What happened?"

"He just . . . went to sleep last night. And then he stopped breathing."

This makes no sense to me. I can hear my mother's grief and bewilderment in her shredded voice; it makes no sense to her, either. He had a cold, she tells me, *just a cold*, which he then gave to her. Around eight or nine, he said that he was tired. He went to bed early in their little guest room, where he'd been sleeping for the past few nights so he wouldn't keep her awake with his coughing. She heard him clear his throat and cough a few times, but then he fell silent, and she assumed he'd finally gotten to sleep. When she went in to check on him later—

"He was so cold."

She said his name, and then she called out for him, and then she shook him. She repeated these steps, over and over. He didn't wake. She called 911, and paramedics arrived within five minutes.

As she speaks, I try to picture the uniformed strangers who tried to save my father; who climbed onto the mattress, pushed up their sleeves, and pushed down on his chest so hard that the wooden slats of the antique bed frame snapped beneath their efforts. They worked diligently, efficiently, taking turns with air and compressions while my mother sobbed and prayed. It will be weeks before it occurs to either of us that Dad had a do-not-resuscitate order in his advance directives, filled out the year before and forgotten in the crisis. When the paramedics stopped, they did so as one, as if they knew, in the same moment, that it was time to let him go. One of them turned to my mother. *I'm sorry. He's gone.*

My parents' priest came to their house and sat up with Mom for the rest of the night. A few friends came to help wash and prepare the body, according to their custom, and then he was taken away. My mother's sister, who had moved to southern Oregon the year I left, came over and began calling family—she'd tried me twice, then left a message. Exhausted, Mom sent everyone home before dawn, knowing that soon the entire parish would know and more people would be arriving to help. She went to lie down, though not to sleep. She couldn't stay upright any longer.

Thousands of miles away, I slept on, beside my silenced phone.

When I ask what I can do, she tells me there is nothing she needs yet. Friends have already brought food, and she is never alone unless she wants to be. She says that the funeral will be on Thursday or Friday; I should start looking for flights. She has to go, some friends want her for something, but she will call me later. I tell her that I love her. There is nothing more to say.

After we hang up, I shout for my husband in a voice I have never used before. I don't know how long I have been crying. Maybe I have been all along. He runs to our room, and I say the words, the words I still can't believe, for the first time.

———

Stable was what my mother would say, when I asked her how he was doing. Dad would tell me that he was *about the same*, or *fine*, or, more commonly, *so wonderful you wish you were me*. Though he relied on my mother for a great deal, he could take care of himself. He'd come through the infection and surgery. His labs had been normal—for him—since then. He wasn't healthy or doing well, we knew that, but I put so much faith in that word, *stable*. Sometimes, when I wanted to reassure myself, I would run through the list, remind myself of all that he was able to do.

He could care for himself during the day when she was at work. Their home and small lot, newly outfitted with wooden ramps built at cost by a contractor friend, were maneuverable for him.

He could get up on his own, shower, get dressed. He liked to wear Hawaiian shirts in the summer, thick sweaters and cardigans in the winter, and hats—baseball or bucket— year-round.

If it was a dialysis day, he would pack his bag of snacks and wait for the medical shuttle to bring him to the treatment center. If not, he might go sit out on the patio, listening to the radio, smoking one of the few cigarettes he still allowed himself, watching the hills change color in the shifting light.

He *puttered around the house*, as my mother put it, taking care of small chores. He couldn't bend over to clean the floors, but he could wash dishes and wipe down the counters. He couldn't manage a lengthy trip to the grocery store, but he could prepare dinner for the two of them.

He was happy to hear from me and chat whenever I called;

unlike my mother, who began lobbing fresh questions as soon as I said I had to go, he knew how to say goodbye and mean it.

He had been on dialysis for six years. I knew he wasn't going to get the long and comfortable life I wanted for him. But I had believed we would get some sort of warning—a bad lab report would come back, I imagined, and the doctor would tell him that dialysis was no longer working. There would come a day when we would know that his death was near. I never imagined that he would simply die, quietly, peacefully, in his sleep.

His death certificate doesn't tell me why. The causes of death are listed as *end-stage renal failure, diabetes mellitus, hypertension*. Yet I have no idea what forced his body to shut down, his heart to stop, on that given night. Was it a cough that gave way to a silent heart attack? Multisystem failure? I will never know for certain. I know more about what did not happen than what did. At no time did he shout for help, or cry out in pain. There was no harsh death rattle, no deep gasps for a final breath he couldn't find. My mother sat not ten feet away from him on the other side of a thin wall, reading a book. If he had called out for her, made any sound of real distress, she would have heard, and gone to him.

When others who loved him tell me I should be thankful that he didn't suffer in the end, a memory rises up, the fragment of a prayer from an Orthodox liturgy I had attended with my parents: *Grant us a peaceful and Christian ending to our lives.* I had been so afraid that he would linger in pain for years, the way I'd been told his mother had. I feared the slow or sudden erosion of his mind or his memory, the day when he would need more care than my mother could provide. She and I had maintained separate and overlapping catalogs of anxieties, worrying that some other malady—dementia, a stroke, a diabetic coma—would befall him, and he would grow less and less like himself: gone, in a sense, before he was really gone. I have just enough of what some would call *perspective* to be glad that none of these things happened, that the moment of death was the peaceful one he'd prayed for. But I cannot be grateful for how he died. He could have lived a hundred years, and my mother and I wouldn't have been ready to let him go.

We don't know the moment he took his last breath, because no one was with him. The time of death I read on the certificate is not the moment his life ended but the moment the paramedics had to give up. I will never know what really happened. I know that he was sick, that he always told me he felt fine, that sometimes he would admit to being tired. That he was alive, and then he wasn't.

He was sixty-seven years old.

———

Many weeks later, a friend calls it *a common American death.* We are in her car, on our way to dinner, speaking of various conditions that run in our families. Both of us have seen our loved ones' health problems exacerbated by financial insecurity, inaccessible medical care. She says that what happened to my father was tragic, and we talk about how it might have been prevented if only he had gotten the help he needed. *How many people here*, she says, *die for the exact same reason every day?*

I think of how many times I have heard terminal illness and death referred to as "equalizers," as if they can flatten our differences and disparities simply because they come for all of us sooner or later. Sickness and grief throw wealthy and poor families alike into upheaval, but they do not transcend the gulfs between us, as some claim——if anything, they often magnify them. Who has the ability to make choices that others lack? Who is left to scramble for piecemeal solutions in an emergency? If you have no rainy-day savings or paid medical leave, if your support system is scant or under-resourced, if preventative or lifesaving treatment is harder for you to access or altogether out of reach, you will have a profoundly different experience from those who become seriously ill——or find themselves caring for sick or dying loved ones—knowing that, if nothing else, they can afford to meet the moment.

This is a country that takes little responsibility for the health and well-being of its citizens while urging us to blame each other—and ourselves—for our precarity under an exploitative system in which all but a small number of us stand to suffer or lose much. A country that first abandons and then condemns people without money who have the temerity to get sick, accusing them of causing their own deaths. It is still hard for me not to think of my father's death as a kind of negligent homicide, facilitated and sped by the state's failure to fulfill its most basic responsibilities to him and others like him. With our broken safety net, our strained systems of care and support, the deep and corrosive inequalities we have yet to address, it's no wonder that so many of us find ourselves alone, struggling to get the help we need when we or our loved ones are suffering.

What killed my father, on paper, was diabetes and kidney failure: common indeed, the eighth- and tenth-leading causes of death in the United States in 2020, according to the Centers for Disease Control. But failing organs, life-threatening infections, death in his sixties—these were not inevitable outcomes, nor matters of pure chance and inheritance, an avalanche of genetic misfortune. He needed access to quality health care in order to manage and treat his illnesses. He needed it throughout his life, not only in his final years, when it was granted as a crisis response only after his kidneys had failed. His mother lived longer and had greater access to life-prolonging treatment in the 1960s and 1970s than her son had in the twenty-first century.

For her part, for reasons I will never comprehend, my mother assigns herself some blame. She knew that he was slowing down. Should she have realized that his death was close? Had she missed important signs? If she had known more, could she have done more for him?

I beg her not to think that way. It's not her fault. She worked so hard to take care of him.

I want to ask if she or Dad blamed me for being so far away. For not being able to help more. I realize that I am afraid to hear the answer, and the question seems too great a burden to add to the ones she already carries. What I feel is not pure self-recrimination—I know his illness wasn't my fault, either. But the regret and anger I bear is a constant ache, fierce and gnawing and deep, so entwined with my grief that I cannot begin to parse where one feeling ends and another begins.

9

AFTER MY FATHER DIED, HIS SISTER ASKED MY MOTHER
when she would be shipping his body "home." Mom was
so confused that she had to repeat the question. My parents
had spent all but the first few years of their married life in
Oregon, and still his family considered Ohio not only Dad's
true home but his final resting place. When Mom told me this
upon my arrival in Oregon, it was the first time I'd laughed,
really laughed, since learning of his death.

There are so many things you do for a person after they
die, things they don't really need—the living do. Rituals,
memorial services, acts of public mourning are all ways of
honoring the person we loved, intended to bring us comfort
as well. I welcomed the chance to work on my father's obitu-
ary, look for photos for the memorial display, find something
suitable for my children to wear to the funeral. I even found
some strange consolation in my attempts to explain the unex-
plainable to them, because these were all duties to manage,

tasks I could do. As long as I had responsibilities, I didn't have to sit with the wrathful stillness of grief.

In the end, however, there were few preparations to throw myself into once I got home, because my parents' friends were already hard at work on their behalf. In their hands, the service and burial would be exactly what my mother wanted. The choir already knew their parts by heart. There was no need to hire a caterer, because everyone was bringing a dish to share. One of the women in the parish was preparing the traditional koliva, a dish of boiled wheat berries, nuts, dried fruits, and seeds painstakingly arranged in a cruciform design, which would be blessed and shared during the mercy meal. Luke, the craftsman who had built my parents' ramps, was working on my father's casket and refused to accept payment for it.

A number of items went into my father's casket to be buried with him: an Orthodox cross, also made of wood and small enough to fit in one of his hands, its three crossbeams lined in thin gold foil; a white cloth draped across his forehead, representing the crown of victory he had earned for running his earthly race, adorned with the prayer *Holy God, Holy Mighty, Holy Immortal, have mercy on us*; an icon of Saint Canice, or Cainnech, his patron saint, a sixth-century Irish abbot who established monasteries and hermitages throughout Ireland and Scotland, for which he is venerated by the Catholic, Orthodox, and Anglican Churches; and an icon of the Ladder of Divine Ascent, a twelfth-century monk's rendering of Saint John Climacus's famous treatise on the thirty steps monastics might progress along in order to reach Christ, who awaits the faithful at the summit, his once-pierced hands outstretched.

———

When I was young, a scholarship kid at a Catholic elementary school who sat through two Masses a week and knew every rite and prayer, it would have been impossible to imagine my parents as anything other than the devout Roman Catholics they'd been ever since a dry, spirited little nun brought them back to the church during their years in Seattle. Yet by the time they left it, in what was less a dramatic sundering than a long, drawn-out farewell, I couldn't be surprised. They had stopped attending our church——the smallest Catholic parish in the area, one that had taken over what used to be a covered farmers' market——around the time I turned sixteen, after years of flirting with Orthodoxy. My mother converted when I was a freshman in college; my father took his time, following her a decade or so later. At the small Orthodox parish where they landed, no one noticed or commented on how often people tithed, as our former priest had; the day he did so was the day my parents, who never had much money to give but faithfully volunteered to run church fundraisers, teach catechism classes, lead Bible studies, began their slow but steady retreat from the church. In their new community, I believe they were seen and known, nurtured and valued, in a way they hadn't been anywhere else. They found communion.

There was no question that my father would have the full Orthodox funeral. My mother told me it was a beautiful liturgy. *We like to joke that it's a reason to convert.* With his siblings unable to travel due to their own health issues, it was his parish family that drew together to mourn and pray for and bury him. I understood why my parents had given their hearts, their prayers, their labor to the little mission church, its altars and rich iconostasis hidden treasures in a rural strip mall, because I could see the joy everyone there took in caring for one another. Witnessing proof of their love for my family also made me wonder what familiar sources of support and comfort I might have given up when I left the small place where I'd been raised, when I was no longer under the know-it-all gazes of neighbors and parishioners who remembered me toddling around in diapers, constantly hailed and questioned by family friends who'd watched me grow up. I couldn't help but compare my parents' tight-knit church, its members' steadfast presence in their lives, with my own distance and relative isolation as their wayward child who rarely made it home.

Before the funeral, parish elders, young parents, children as young as five and six approached, red-eyed or weeping, to tell me how much they had loved my father. We stood together over his body—which I could not think of as *him*—resting in the handsome casket his friend had made, with its clean lines and dark walnut stain, no adornments save a small wooden Orthodox cross painted gold and set on the lid. As happens at all open-casket funerals, everyone told my mother that Dad looked really good for being dead.

"They did a great job on him," she agreed.

"We should all look so good when we enter the Kingdom!" someone exclaimed.

During the service, my parents' friend and former priest,

the one who'd anointed my mother at her Chrismation, talked about my father with great respect and affection. He said he always felt that Dad loved people *beyond their merits*, a sentiment to which I could relate; while Dad and I sometimes disappointed each other, our love was never in question, and he usually thought better of me than I thought of myself. Their current parish priest spoke of the daily pain Dad had lived with and how, in the end, he'd allowed this suffering to bring him closer and closer to the God he would soon meet. This, the priest concluded, is why my father ultimately knew peace at his death: it did not find him unready. He was intimately familiar with his body's weaknesses, his own mortality, and had used his suffering to focus his mind and prepare his soul.

Of course, he couldn't know the day or the hour. But he knew he would soon meet our Lord, and he prepared for that meeting.

I couldn't have been more surprised if the priest had walked over and slapped me, though years of church training helped me hold the line. I supposed he could speak with some authority when it came to my father's true feelings about faith, life, and death—he had pastored him, counseled him, heard his confessions for years—but if what he said was true, why had he seen it when my mother and I had not? Had Dad truly spent the past weeks, maybe even months, preparing to die? If he'd known it was imminent, why didn't he warn my mother? Why didn't he tell me, his only child, so I could try to say goodbye? I stared at my father in his handmade casket, and the sudden flare of anger I felt was so unlike sorrow that I let myself take momentary refuge in it. *If you really knew and didn't tell us, that was a real dick move, Dad.*

He did look peaceful, as if he had welcomed death, or

at least been ready for it. When we approached to say our final goodbyes, Mom, mostly cried out by then, put her arm around my shoulders, her solid warmth a familiar comfort as always.

"Don't despair," she told me. "This is our hope in the Resurrection."

The words might have upset me coming from anyone else in that church, anyone else in the world. But I felt her sorrow as something deeper and more powerful than my own, a great river spilling its banks. I couldn't help but feel awed by her abiding faith in what she saw as my father's victory over death. She was a warrior, even in grief.

Though it was the middle of winter, she had asked that the traditional Paschal Troparion be sung at his grave. Everyone in attendance took a turn with the shovel, dropping earth over his casket with the Easter song of triumph resounding in our ears:

> *Christ is risen from the dead,*
> *trampling down death by death,*
> *and upon those in the tombs bestowing life.*

I was no longer a regular Sunday Mass goer. There were too many things that I felt ambivalent about or disagreed with altogether, though when I did make it to church, I still found some reassurance in the rhythm of the liturgy, the prayers I'd known since childhood, the echo of moments when I'd felt a whisper of something like grace. I knew it would always be a link to my parents and how they raised me; now, if I wanted, I could go to Mass and try to believe what I had been taught—that I was touching eternity while earthbound, in communion with my father and everyone I would ever love or lose.

As I get older, I've found there are some answers I don't need. I can't say whether I'll ever again feel as certain of anything as my parents were of the prevailing mercy of God or the promise of heaven. But it's also true that the faith you're raised in can still move fathoms below the surface, even when your relationship to it has changed beyond recognition. As I held my mother's hand, watching my father's casket disappear beneath a layer of earth, perhaps I shouldn't have been surprised to feel the old belief stir, bearing me up like a strong current, as undeniable as it was unseen.

———

After my mother joined the Orthodox Church, I think my father was less inclined than she to commit his time and energy to another religion that might not deserve it. But their shared faith had long been the bedrock of their marriage, and eventually Mom got tired of going to liturgy alone. She knew that Dad had no theological objections to Orthodoxy, and thought he was being ornery, or lazy; no doubt he did enjoy staying home most Sundays, especially during football season. Finally, she lost patience. *You need to find some church that'll bury you when the time comes, you know.* When he started regularly attending liturgy with her, I think it was less because he took this foreboding line to heart, and more that he felt a renewed hunger for religious discipline and community. My parents were alike in their desire to believe in something, to own that belief as an absolute guiding truth. They had always seen God at work in their lives, in our family—in my adoption, especially.

On one of my father's first Sundays at the parish, he halted at the entrance, causing my mother to run into him and ask what he'd seen. He pointed to an icon above the door, one of dozens that filled the walls. "I've seen that before!"

It was an icon of the Ladder of Divine Ascent. Mom, a recent but fervent devotee of iconography, started to explain its provenance, the story of Saint John Climacus and his Ladder of Paradise, but Dad interrupted. "I don't mean I've seen the icon before. I mean, I've seen *that ladder*. I saw it right after we moved here."

She stared at him. "What are you talking about?"

After my parents moved to Oregon, they would often spend their days off driving with no particular destination in mind, exploring and getting to know the area. One afternoon they were heading home from somewhere far out in the country, the region's tallest Cascadian volcano in full view, when my father suddenly glimpsed a ladder beside it, partially hidden by clouds encircling the peak. If he squinted, he could see tiny figures clinging to the rungs, some slowly ascending while others stumbled and fell as if attacked, pulled down by unseen forces. He watched in wonder for a few seconds, but when he blinked, the ladder and everyone climbing it disappeared.

He didn't have an explanation for what he'd seen, couldn't begin to guess what it meant, so he never told anyone. Not until some thirty years later when, entering a mission church housed in a storefront, he encountered an icon written by a long-dead monk at a monastery on Mount Sinai. "That's what I saw on the mountain when we were driving home all those years ago," he said to my mother, who was still looking at him in astonishment. "That's my ladder."

———

Written for monastics and studied for centuries by laypeople as well, Saint John Climacus's *Ladder of Divine Ascent* is one of the most influential religious texts ever written, an allegorical model of the Christian journey to holiness. The thirty rungs of his ladder represent thirty steps: passions to be mastered, vices to conquer, virtues to attain in pursuit of true union with God. Among the virtues extolled is remembrance of death, which "produces the putting aside of cares and constant prayer and guarding of the mind."

John Climacus wasn't suggesting anyone should wish for death, and took care to distinguish between a "natural" and a "contranatural" preoccupation with it—the remembrance of death, he asserted, should inspire us to live as God would wish and do as much good as we can. But he also urged the faithful to foster what he saw as a healthy detachment from earthbound cares and concerns, so as not to permit the struggles and sufferings of this life to compromise one's readiness for the next. "Just as the Fathers lay down that perfect love is free from falls," he wrote, "so I for my part declare that a perfect sense of death is free from fear . . . It is impossible, someone says, impossible to spend the present day devoutly unless we regard it as the last of our whole life." It's a charge that reminds me of the old Ash Wednesday exhortation, recited as crosses are drawn on Catholics' foreheads: *Remember, man, you are dust, and to dust you shall return.* In the Christian sense, these are calls to repentance, but they can also be read as invitations to surrender: to accept our limitations and our mortality; to be prepared, not consumed with clawing fear, for our life's eventual end; to focus on doing good and not harm, because any day could be our last.

After my father's death, my mother told me she believed that he often perceived things she could not. She said he was more able to grasp certain matters at an instinctive level, to accept them on faith, whereas she was always quick to question or feel frustrated by that which she could not immediately understand, whether it was theology or algebra or decisions made by people she loved. I know this was true within the little triumvirate of our family—Dad would storm when he lost his temper, but he tended to recover quickly; Mom often found it harder to move past hurt feelings after an argument—so perhaps it also proved true amid everything my father endured in his final months. My mother railed against his illnesses, resented them, as you do when someone you love is in pain. I know my father struggled as well, and maybe at times even despaired, but I think he must have at least begun to move beyond the point where physical suffering ruled his every mood, consumed his every thought. Of the three of us, at least, he was the quickest to make peace with what would happen.

He had to have been feeling his worst before he died, yet when we spoke, he didn't lash out, as he sometimes had in the past when he was in pain. He sounded so calm and peaceful in our last few phone calls that I could almost forget how much he was enduring. I couldn't understand it after he died, of course, but then I am much more like my mother: I hated Dad's sickness and his pain, blamed myself for not being able to help, resented the God in whose "plan" I was told to trust for not helping him, yet could never manage to convince myself that he would die. If he *had* told me he was about to die but did not dread it—because he was "remembering death," because God was calling him, or because he had somehow found strength in something far beyond his own pain and fear—I would not have wanted to hear him. I would have begged him to seek help and fight. I would have denied him that peace until the end.

A belief echoed throughout Eastern and Western Christian traditions is that suffering, both spiritual and physical, is no meaningless, quotidian component of life, an unfortunate reality that all of us must endure since our fall from grace; rather, it's held that suffering can be purposeful, even redemptive, a route to Christ for those who seek him. No cradle Catholic raised by parents like mine can forget being taught that in suffering we find kinship with all who suffer, communion with the God who suffered for our sake. But it's not a lesson I have learned particularly well. I am still so afraid of suffering, afraid of death—even that "peaceful" death, the kind we are supposed to want, to pray for; the kind my father supposedly experienced.

What wouldn't I do to prevent my own suffering, and the suffering of those I love—my children, my husband, my mother? What ineffable, unknowable graces wouldn't I have denied my father, if I could have brought an end to his pain through some means other than the silent, holy death I'm told he had?

If he did know that he was close to dying, maybe our refusal to accept his suffering, accept what it meant, accept the inevitable, is why he didn't see fit to tell us. Or maybe, my mother later theorized, laughing and crying at once, he wanted to spare us the knowledge: *It might have been the one truly noble act of his life.*

By then, I was afraid of losing her, too. I didn't know what to believe. I still don't know what I *want* to believe. In my memory, my father wasn't prone to hiding the truth in order to comfort others. But neither was he prone to visions. Was it really there, the ladder he saw that day, propped up against the snowcapped summit? Of course it wasn't. I am sure that he imagined it. But I can't claim to know what it means that he did.

10

GRIEF COMES IN WAVES, EVERYONE SAYS. AFTER MY FA-
ther's death, I kept waiting to be buffeted, swept under. I was
sure that his loss was all I would be able to feel once the shock
began to ebb.

In the days leading up to his funeral, I carried the knowledge that he was gone in my tight chest, my aching throat,
my stomach that felt as though I'd swallowed a riverbed's
worth of stones. I both feared and hoped that traveling home,
seeing my mother, would allow my grief to flow more freely.
But we hadn't yet landed in Oregon when I became aware of
a pervasive everyday frustration boiling beneath the sorrow.
The flights were long and stressful, and our nine-year-old
kept looking either surly or sick when we tried to talk with
her—loquacious since toddlerhood, suddenly she was limit-
ing herself to one-word, irritable answers, shaking her head
when we asked a question or expressed concern. Her little
sister, usually a good traveler, was likewise short-tempered
and clingy.

Their moods did not improve once we arrived. Though Dan did his best to manage them, trying to spare me further strain, I was aware every time the kids fussed or fought, wavering between vexation and worry. It wasn't their fault, I tried to tell myself—how were they supposed to know what to do with death at their ages? I was nearly a decade into parenting; I should be accustomed to putting aside my own feelings and needs when necessary. But the sight of my mother trying to cheer up her cranky grandchildren the night before she buried her husband made me feel raw and resentful, and I began to wish that I had left the rest of my family at home. At least then I would have been able to focus on my mother, and she wouldn't be forced to placate my children instead of attending to her own grief.

I texted my friends: *There is no room at all for my feelings with the kids here*. They were all sympathetic, but they reminded me that it was important for my children to be there. *Even if they weren't super close to your dad, it's their first experience with death. They need to be able to witness it and say goodbye*. I knew this was true. Still, I kept wishing that I could be cared for, instead of having to be a caregiver. I didn't want to have to be a parent while I buried my father; I only wanted to be a grieving daughter.

———

Later, when someone asked me about my father's funeral, I said, "It was beautiful. My mother was really happy with how it went. And my sister was there with me, which was so kind of her."

The person nodded, looking a little confused. *Wouldn't your sister be there?* their expression seemed to say.

"Oh," I said, "no. I'm adopted. My dad wasn't her dad. Ah, but we do have the same parents."

I met my sister, Cindy, when I was twenty-seven and she was thirty-three. In another life, if our parents had made other choices, we would have grown up together. As it was, she hadn't even known I was alive when I made contact with my birth family in the same month my first child was born. I couldn't have predicted that she and her family would become such a steadfast source of love and support, the kind many people don't get from relatives they've known all their lives. It has now been fourteen years since we found each other—since our correspondence began, and those first careful, hopeful letters gave way to one visit, then many more. My kids have known their aunt Cindy all their lives, but I understand how easily they might never have known her at all, and have told them the story of what we did to put part of our family back together. When I see my sister, talk with her, it feels as if we are recovering lost treasure. In her company, I'm able to be my whole self.

She and her husband, Rick, had met my adoptive parents only once before. Yet when my father died, they both took time off work to make the five-hour drive from Portland, arriving just in time to help and offer my children the crucial distraction of a cousin to play with. Cindy and I cleaned my mother's house so it would be ready for visitors. My brother-in-law ran errands, took the kids to the playground, picked up dinner for all of us.

On the morning of the funeral, Dan and I had to call the girls three times before they would stop giggling with their cousin and change into their church clothes. I was worried we would be late, but it was good to see them smiling and looking like themselves again. I inspected them in their dresses and sweaters and buckled leather flats, adjusted their wavy brown ponytails. Again, I tried to explain what was about to happen, though I hardly believed it myself.

"We're going to Grandma's church to pray, and then we'll go to the cemetery to bury Grandpa. You'll get to see him and say goodbye."

The sudden shock of my father's death was difficult for either of our children to comprehend. Our younger daughter, who had turned seven a few days earlier, found it hardest to grapple with the abstract yet absolute finality of death due to her age and, perhaps, her autism. While she had seen movies and read books touching on death, it was not yet a solid concept to her. Dan and I had tried to explain what it *meant* that her grandpa was gone—that she wouldn't see him again as she had known him, and that we were all very sad and would miss him—but these conversations felt no easier, even after several attempts. I wasn't sure how to bridge the space between our words and her understanding of what had happened when I was still struggling to absorb it myself.

When we brought our children up to the casket to see my father one last time, tears were drifting down our older daughter's cheeks. I took her hand, then put my arm around her and drew her close, as my mother had done with me. My younger daughter reached out, hesitantly, and touched my father's gray beard. Her fingers brushed his cold cheek. She smiled down at him, just a little smile.

"Goodbye, Grandpa. We love you. We'll miss you."

I was, and had been for years now, more mother than daughter. It occurred to me that this was one thing about me my dad would have understood, because he, too, was more parent and partner than dutiful son. He hadn't been able to visit his family in Ohio as often as they wanted. While he had worked hard for as long as he could, work was never his life, nor, I think, central to how he defined himself. He'd left everything he knew behind to start a new life with my mother, and then with me: we were his life. Perhaps he had not blamed me for living on the other side of the country, or focusing on my kids and their needs, because he understood the life I'd chosen when I became a parent.

There are no shortcuts when it comes to helping your children understand what it means to love people who will die, and to live with that knowledge. Seeing my father in his casket, touching his face, registering that he wasn't getting up to make one of his silly jokes to get her to laugh—these experiences are what allowed my younger child to understand what had happened to him and to our family. She would refer to this moment for weeks, for years, in conversations about her grandpa; it would stay with her, make his loss believable, where all of our well-meaning words had fallen short. Maybe it was okay, I thought, that I didn't know exactly what to say to my daughters—how to translate this loss for them, put my terrible grief into words. We were here now, missing my dad, saying goodbye. We were learning what that meant together.

—

My mother invited Cindy and Rick back to the house after the funeral and reception, and we all sat around talking, watching the three cousins chase each other around and record goofy videos together. Mom grinned and shook her head, aiming a good-natured lecture or two in their direction, and I could see that this was good for her. I understood that my sister and her husband hadn't come to stand in the place of our absent family; they were with us now because they *were* our family. I'd known they were mine, of course, and I'd known I could count on them; I just hadn't realized that their love and care for me could be extended so easily, so generously, to my mom. It was a scene like nothing I could have imagined when I was growing up adopted. What did these generous, openhearted people have in common? Only their love for me.

The conversation turned to my soon-to-be-published debut book, about my adoption and the search for my Korean family. My brother-in-law kicked it off by marveling that I'd summed him up in a sentence. My sister said that reading the book made her feel as if she knew my dad a little better, and she was happy that she got to meet him before he died. My mom, for her part, said she had been glad to learn more about my birth family. Dan chimed in that he was proud of me, and the kids wanted to know when they would be allowed to read it. I was mostly quiet, listening to them talk about the various curiosities and connections between us. I felt my dad's absence, but also his love, stronger than ever.

In my birth family, I remain a ghost to this day. My birth parents told their relatives that I died as a baby, and this is still what nearly all of them believe. Most of my living Korean relatives wouldn't recognize me if they saw me. I cannot say whether my ancestors would heed me if I asked for their protection. But I know the parents who raised me, the sister who reclaimed me. I am grateful that I was able to bring them together, if only briefly.

At the end of the day, my mom hugged my sister and her husband, thanking them for being there for my father's funeral. For all of us. "Of course," my sister said. "You're our family now, too." I don't remember which of the three said they hoped we'd all get the chance to be together again. But I found myself hoping for the same.

11

THERE WAS A MOMENT, BEFORE MY HUSBAND, KIDS, AND I left for my father's funeral, when I had to make our excuses to a fellow parent. My younger daughter had been invited to her child's birthday party. I texted to explain that she would miss the party, and why. *I'm sorry, Nicole*, she wrote back. *It's so hard to lose a parent. But it will be a comfort to see your father live on in your children.*

I stared at the screen for a moment, uncomprehending, until the meaning of her words sank in. *She doesn't know that I'm adopted.*

At some point you learn that the purpose of life, for most creatures on the planet, is to pass on their genes before they die. In seventh-grade biology class, our teacher—who had a PhD, a species of beetle named after him, and a deep philosophical streak—said that this was the only form of immortality accessible to most of the living: we would die, but if we had children, and they had children, our genes, the essence of who we are and everything that makes us *us*, would live on.

Even back then, I remember thinking about how that wasn't going to work out for my parents.

They were never going to see glimpses of themselves in me or in my children. When my father was alive, I know he sometimes struggled to see himself in me, too. We were different in such undeniable ways, most of which had nothing to do with the genes determining the pigment of our skin, the shape of our eyes. He was always embarrassing me, laughing or cracking jokes when I most wanted to be serious, trying out his impromptu stand-up routine on my friends when he drove us to the mall or the movie theater. He'd watch me tapping away at a keyboard, or writing in my notebook until my hand cramped up, and it was as foreign to him as his love of football was to me. He did not understand my obsession with my grades. He did not understand my career. We rarely voted the same way, and he couldn't resist telling me whenever he believed that I was wrong.

I know that my father loved me, and I know he was proud of me: How many people need and deserve such assurance from a parent and never get it? But sometimes I did not know how to respond when he got angry. I have always been stubborn to a fault; the more someone screams, the less likely I am to back down. Once, I asked him to change the television channel because the program he was watching struck me as too violent for my then eight- and five-year-old kids, who were playing nearby, to see. He ignored me, I asked again, and he shouted that I was *full of shit*, threw the remote at me, and stalked out of the room. It was my children's shocked and anxious expressions that lit my own fuse—I followed him down the hall to his room, yelling that he couldn't speak to me that way anymore, especially in front of them. He turned his face to the wall, refusing to look at me. There was nothing to do about it, my mother said. *You know how your father is.*

My parents would often tell me that their love was all the greater because of my adoption. *We* chose *you*, they would remind me. *You were meant to be ours.* I've never doubted their love, but sometimes I have wondered if my adoption added just a little more anxious weight to our disagreements and disparities, made us all feel a little less secure, in some hard and often unspeakable way. I know that when I've been most upset with them, or they with me, I have felt they couldn't possibly have adopted someone they understood less. And I'm sure they must have had similar, unwelcome thoughts about me in frustration, or fury, or plain confusion. One of my most vivid childhood memories is my mother telling me, *We weren't prepared to have a kid like you.* She didn't say it in anger. She sounded more perplexed than anything else.

I could never entirely rule out adoption as a factor when we fought, or failed to understand one another. There was never any question that we would make up, mend whatever rifts might exist. Still, when what ties you to one another is not blood or birth or even mutual choice, but a piece of paper and a proclamation that you are family—when you haven't always belonged to one another, and can imagine countless scenarios in which you would have remained strangers, never to meet—*is* there more vulnerability, perhaps more to fear, when some emotional or physical distance opens up between you? When you fight, and those bonds are pulled and tested? When one of you is gone forever?

—

The final manuscript of my first book, *All You Can Ever Know*, was due to my publisher two days after my father died. I'm sure I could have gotten an extension. But I couldn't abide the thought of the book hanging over me at his funeral, or in the weeks to follow, and I was afraid I'd never complete it if I allowed myself a pause. The full weight of grief felt so close, an aching heaviness in my chest, an unformed shadow in my peripheral vision that I could not quite see or lay hands on yet. I knew it would soon run me down—I might be a day or two, perhaps only hours, away from falling apart—and so, in the strange, disbelieving lull I now know was shock, I sat down at my kitchen table, tried to wall off every feeling, every part of my brain that wasn't occupied by the book, and pushed through my final revisions while Dan did laundry and packed our bags.

You "finish" a book many times before it's finished. I had completed the rough draft a couple months before my father died, and held on to it for a few craven weeks before sending it to my parents the week of Thanksgiving. I knew they needed to read it; I knew that I needed their honest reactions, whatever they were. I heard nothing for a month.

"I know you're really busy," I finally ventured, "but it's not *War and Peace*?"

My mother explained that it was slow going because she would often read my book aloud to my father, the two of them working their way through it together, chapter by chapter, in the quiet evening interlude between dinner and Dad's early bedtime. When he tried to read the manuscript on his own, he needed a magnifying glass to see the words in twelve-point Times. He died before they could reach the end. Many weeks later, my mother would finish it on her own.

My parents always encouraged my writing—maybe not at two in the morning, or eleven thirty on a school night, but in principle—even if they didn't understand where the urge to write came from. I'm sure they didn't know what they were in for when I began begging for bargain packs of spiral notebooks and boxes of Paper Mate pens; they were probably just glad that my creative obsession was so easily and cheaply fed. The journals and notebooks that piled up in my room were followed by a string of old electric typewriters and secondhand computers that could barely run a word processing program without crashing. Sometimes I deigned to show my family my stories; more often, they read them without my permission. I was better at hiding my diary, but my mother always found it eventually. No matter how many hours my parents might have spent wondering and watching me write, I'm willing to bet they didn't give much thought to the notion that I might one day publish a memoir. I never quoted Czesław Miłosz to them—*When a writer is born into a family, the family is finished*—though I was tempted to do so, once or twice, as a joke.

Of course, I wasn't born into our family at all—a fact that always mattered more to me than it did to them. They saw my adoption as God's handiwork, and therefore above questioning. This was a perspective I understood, but eventually could no longer share. As I grew older, I came to see my adoption as the way I joined my family; the most obvious explanation, if not the only one, for our many differences; the source of questions I would need a lifetime to understand. When the simple story I'd always known was no longer enough for me, when I began to reconsider what I'd been told about my origins and search for a far more complicated, long-buried truth, my parents did their best to listen and to support me. And yet for all the conversations we had about what was lost and gained through adoption—for all my certainty that it was never a single event in my past, but an ongoing, living story to be continually reckoned with—I had not considered how my experiences as an adoptee would tint the edges of my grief when I began to lose them.

———

On the one hand, writing is in my genes: my birth father is also a writer, and our family has nearly always had at least one writer or scholar in each generation, even at times when sending any children to school was a hardship. But sometimes I wonder if I would have become a writer were I not an adoptee. All my life, or at least as long as I have been able to speak for myself, I have had to decide whether and how to meet people's questions about my family; I have been a teacher and a translator and a storyteller, even when I might not have wished to be. I think, too, that being adopted is partly what made me search for new words to express who I was, to make sense of what I saw, to build new worlds to escape to.

When I began writing *All You Can Ever Know*, I told my parents about my plans. They were happy for me, if also a bit surprised. "You're not famous," my mother said. "Do you think anyone is going to read it?" I asked if she minded the idea of my writing the story of my adoption, and she told me she didn't, though she added, half-joking, that I should "only say nice things" about our family.

It's daunting work, turning the people you love into characters in a story—not to reduce or shortchange them, but to try to make them come alive on the page so that other people will understand them, too, and see a little of what you see in them. When my parents told me that they had read the first half of my book and thought it was "good, so far," the relief I felt was overwhelming. I'd been worried that they would dispute my memories, tell me *that's not what happened*. Instead, they lauded my memory, praised the writing. "It's exciting, like a novel, except it's the truth," Mom said. Dad was thrilled that a terrible old joke—his standard reply to nosy people who asked my parents how our family had come to be—made it into the manuscript. *If you put a Pole and a Hungarian together, you get a Korean. Where do you think they all came from?* When I called home on Christmas, he told me, "It's not the story your mom or I would have written about your life. But that's okay. The point is, it's *your* life. It's based on your memories of what happened to you. And I think it's a great Christmas present."

Two weeks later, he was gone.

I cannot remember my last conversation with him. When I called home in his final months, I would often catch him on his own while my mother was at work. Later, if Mom asked him what we'd chatted about, all he would tell her was that we'd had a good talk. This is my sense of those calls as well, although no particular one stands out in my memory. My mother later said that our weekday talks had represented a turning point for him.

"He knew that he wasn't doing well," she told me. "I think he decided that it was time to accept you, love you, forgive you for everything—and just be your father."

If that is true, he must have made the decision during his final weeks, the weeks my parents spent reading my book together. There was nothing in it that I hadn't already discussed with them—by then, we had all learned how to talk about my adoption in ways we couldn't when I was young. But giving them my book to read meant sharing in new, expanded language who I had become, how I differed from them, what it had been like to be their adopted child, without mitigation or platitudes. They could have resented me for it, or felt threatened by the many ways in which my feelings and experiences diverged from theirs. Instead, their response was *We see you*. While I wish that I could recall the last thing my father said to me, I find some solace in allowing his appreciation for the story I labored over—one in which I tried to explore and honor both the truth of my adoption and my adoptive parents' love for me—to stand in for the final words I don't remember.

12

AFTER MY FATHER DIES, I BECOME, FOR A TIME, SOMEONE
I do not recognize. Entire weeks are all but lost to me, scooped
out of my once-airtight memory. Our rental term ends two
months after the funeral, and when we move into another
house, our third residence in seven years, I will hardly remember packing or unpacking.

I don't know how to ask for leave from my job. I tell myself that I can't afford to take unpaid time off anyway. The
truth is that I have always been able to work, and now I learn
that grief is no hindrance to my productivity. I bank on this,
even feel a kind of twisted pride in it. It doesn't matter to me
whether I take care of myself, because I do not deserve the
care. All my parents ever wanted was to spend more time with
us, to see us more than once a year or every other year, and
I never found a way to make it happen, and now my father is
dead. When other people—my husband, my friends—try to
tell me that I am not at fault, I barely hear them. Punishing
myself, keeping myself in as much pain as possible, seems like

something a good daughter should do if it is too late for her to do anything else.

There is a flurry of activity in the run-up to the publication of my first book. My publisher sends me to trade conferences, schedules readings and interviews. I am grateful, and frankly surprised, to be getting any attention at all, and so of course I tell everyone that I am more than ready to do my part, to help the book succeed. I know how important it is to my career, and I feel enormous pressure not to let down any of the people who are working so hard on it. I want it to have a fighting chance, too, because it is a book in which my father still lives.

When I stop working, it's not to rest but to head to a soccer game or swimming lesson, or plan a Girl Scout meeting, or meet with my younger daughter's special educator, or chaperone a school field trip. I treat myself like a machine, which makes it easy for the people I work and volunteer with in various capacities to see and treat me that way, too. "It's been hard," I say with a shrug, when asked how I'm doing, "but I'm hanging in there." One day, after we run into some friends in the neighborhood, my older child calls me out on my usual choice of words.

"How come you always tell people that you're 'hanging in there'?" she asks.

Well, I think, a bit defensively, *because I* am. Am I not still doing what needs to be done: getting up every morning and going to work, taking care of my family, saying yes to anything anyone asks me to do? I haven't dropped a single ball at work. My publishing team has thanked me for my promptness in replying to their emails, for being *so great to work with.* I am an expert at grieving under capitalism. Watch and learn.

All the while, I keep daydreaming about walking into traffic.

From the moment the thought pushes its way into my grief-muddled brain, I know that I could never act on it. It's not that I want to hurt myself—it's that I cannot seem to work up any remorse when I think about no longer being alive. Nor does the thought frighten me, as it always did before. *What if you didn't have to feel this way anymore?* my mind proposes, in moments that are deceptively calm, moments when I am not sobbing in the shower or screaming in my car because I cannot scream at home. *What if the pain could just end?*

As a child, I knew that I was not permitted to indulge in the hyperbolic or sarcastic statements other kids made about wanting to die, because my father would erupt. Toward the end of sixth grade, my teacher had everyone in my class write a fake will; my most charitable reading is that the exercise might have been intended to help us identify the things that were most important to us as we moved from elementary into middle school, symbolically leaving our childhoods behind. Most of my classmates made light of the task—*I hereby bequeath my Game Boy to my little brother, because he always steals it anyway*—but I remember little of what I wrote in my will, only my father's fury over the assignment. "You're twelve years old!" he yelled. He threatened to call my teacher. And then all the fight went out of him, his voice numb as he told me about being twenty-one years old and witnessing the death of his favorite cousin. The two of them had shared an apartment in a Cleveland high-rise, and one night my father came home to find him about to jump from their window. He pleaded with him, tried to stop him, but his cousin leaped before he could reach him. Dad had always blamed himself.

It takes me months, after his death, to realize that I am not *fine*, or *hanging in there*. I go to see my primary care doctor for a long-overdue physical and break down in the exam room, sobbing as she hands me one flimsy tissue after another. I leave with a referral to a counseling practice, but manage to find one even closer to my house, close enough to walk, because I know that I'll come up with a million reasons to reschedule or cancel unless it's practically in the neighborhood.

During one early session, my therapist, the first Asian American therapist I have ever worked with, asks me if I know what has kept me from harming myself as I flounder in grief. I don't even have to think about the answer. "My family," I say. My children, who have no idea how dark my thoughts have become. My husband, who keeps our household afloat on days when I cannot manage anything beyond the workday. My sister, who faithfully checks on me every week. My mother, whom I text and call so often it probably annoys her. "The people I love still need me."

"And you still need them," she says. "You don't want to leave them."

I feel the truth of these words in my bones, try to keep them close as the weeks go by.

Not all at once, but slowly, I find my footing again. When I catch myself faltering, fumbling in the dark for a thread to follow back to the person I was before, the thing that often keeps me from despair is talking with my mother. Sometimes

I wish that she would voice some concrete need, ask me to do something for her, but she seems to be taking care of herself—it occurs to me that this might be easier than taking care of both herself and Dad, as much as she misses him. I can sense her sorrow and restlessness, always, but there is a driving, don't-quit vitality about her, even in mourning. I feel certain she has never doubted, for a second, that living is worth it.

One day, she tells me that she has decided to get rid of Dad's lift chair, and one of their old end tables. *I never liked that table, Dad did. I am learning that I can make decisions based on what I want—that if I don't like something, I can just make a change, or do something differently.* Another day, we discuss whether she might get a dog; it has been a long time since she had one in the house. She sheepishly tells me that she used some of the money I gave her to buy new mini blinds. "That's perfect!" I say. I don't care how she spends it, as long as it's useful.

It's hard for either of us to imagine her remarrying, or wanting to remarry. But as she begins to plan the next stage of her life without my father, I realize that I can picture her living out her own days in peace—and, more important, it seems that she can as well. My heart lifts when she tells me that she is planning a trip to Greece with two of her friends from church, intending to use what's left of my father's life insurance payout to make her first-ever trip outside the country. All our calls are filled with talk of her plans: She and her friends are hoping to travel in the fall. They will visit monasteries and holy sites, see the sights, and swim in the sea; the trip is to be part pilgrimage, part escape. Her passport has long since expired, but she's started the renewal process.

After that adventure—once she's ready—I resolve to help her consider what she wants her new life to look like. At least I can be her sounding board, if nothing else. I know her ties to Oregon are strong after four decades there—there's her church, her chosen family, and I doubt she would consider leaving the area as long as my grandmother still lives there—but maybe someday she'll decide that she wants to move closer to us. Or maybe we can relocate to the Northwest and provide more support to her once our kids are done with school. There's no need to figure everything out now, I tell myself. Dad has been gone only a matter of months. Mom has time.

We have time.

13

I WAS READING CONGRATULATORY TEXTS FROM FRIENDS and hadn't even made it out of bed when my mother called me on my publication day. She had seen her doctor the day before to discuss some mysterious spotting. A scan had revealed a strange mass in her abdomen, and now her doctor was referring her to a surgeon to have it removed and sent for testing. Mom was already convinced of the worst.

"What if it's cancer?" she said, her voice low and choked with fear.

We had buried Dad nine months earlier. I would not allow myself to imagine anything happening to her. "You had a hysterectomy twenty years ago," I said, as if she needed to be reminded. "You don't have any organs there where cancer could develop. It's got to be benign."

Over the next few weeks, my book tour took me all over the country: Seattle, Austin, Boston, New York. I would stop at home long enough to reconnect with my family, unpack, and have my event clothes dry-cleaned, then take off with another suitcase stuffed with dresses and jumpsuits. No matter where I was, my mother always knew the forecast. "You're supposed to be having beautiful fall weather in Boston," she'd say when I called; or, "Did you arrive before or after the big storm in Chicago?" I realized that she was tracking my travels in weather systems as a way of looking after me.

I was able to stop in Oregon to see her before her surgery. A bookstore one town over offered to host me for a reading; she drove us there and sat in the front row. My high school guidance counselor was in attendance, as were my beloved second-grade teacher and a friend who'd made her husband drive ninety minutes so she could be there. When an audience member asked me if my adoptive parents were "offended" by anything I'd written, Mom sat up a bit straighter in her chair and said loudly, "*No.*" After I finished my talk, she asked one of the booksellers if she could have the promotional poster they'd placed in the window.

"A real mom power move," I said with a laugh.

"Well, it's a nice picture of you!" she said. "I'm very proud of you, hon. Your dad is, too."

Her surgeon was optimistic following the outpatient procedure, reporting that the tumor wasn't large and that she had gotten everything she could see and taken margins for further testing. A few days later I was at a book festival, about to head to my first event of the day, when Mom texted me with the results: stage 2 cancer. *Ovarian, endometrial, it's hard to know exactly what to call it.* She sounded exhausted and overwhelmed when I reached her on the phone, much as she had in the last years of my dad's life, and I hated hearing those familiar notes in her voice. She said that I should talk to her surgeon to get all the details, and gave me her number.

I remember almost nothing I said during the festival panel, held onstage beneath stained-glass windows in a church filled to capacity. Later that afternoon, between a reading at a museum and a live radio interview, I was able to reach the surgeon. She was kind and direct; I could see why my mother liked her. Based at a research hospital in Portland, she frequently traveled to more rural areas to consult with local gynecology and oncology practices on "the really tricky cases," or so Mom had said.

"I have never seen a situation quite like this before," she admitted. "I think, because of your mother's severe endometriosis, it was not possible for the surgeon who performed her hysterectomy years ago to take everything out; a few fragments were left, and that is where the cancer grew. This tumor looks very similar to ovarian cancer, and it's where her ovaries used to be, so that is how we will treat it. Your mother joked that I might get an interesting paper out of this."

Yes, I thought. *That sounds like her.*

We were thankful when the other tissue tests came back clear, showing no sign of any remaining cancer. My mother's oncologist recommended that she undergo chemotherapy "just to be sure," but the prognosis, we were both assured, was excellent. Her treatments would be covered by Medicare, which she had just qualified for based on age, sparing her one worry, at least—there was no mountain of medical debt waiting on the other side of this crisis.

"The doctors said that after this I should be cured," she told me.

She sounded surprised. I understood why. After she'd recovered from breast cancer, her doctors had steadfastly avoided using that word; they would say that she was in re-mission, or that there was no further evidence of disease. Many years passed before they would pronounce her "cured."

Three months later, she had another clean scan, and her oncologist said as much again: she was cured. Grateful though she was, she still wondered at the phrase. "I didn't think they usually said that about cancer," she said. "I sure hope they're right."

———

She flew out to visit us in August, a few months after finishing chemo, toting two giant suitcases. One of them was stuffed with gifts for the kids—watercolors and markers, notebooks and pens, modeling clay and a package of multicolored sand. The three of them made enormous messes at the picnic table on the patio. I have a picture from one of those afternoons: my mom beaming in a peach-colored embroidered T-shirt, looking well despite having lost a dress size to chemo, her close-cropped hair growing back, happy to be bookended by her granddaughters. It was hot and humid, the air flecked with bugs, but she was content to sit in the dappled shade of our Kwanzan cherry tree, reading one of the mystery novels she'd brought with her or chatting with the kids while they played. She spent many hours watching my younger daughter, the only one of us who didn't seem to mind the heat, soar back and forth on the circular swing we'd hung from a tree branch, her joy a palpable thing as she twisted in flight.

Toward the end of her visit, Mom poked her head into my office and asked, "Do you have any Kotex?" Her preferred brand, and what she called all menstrual pads, the way some people refer to any brand of facial tissues as Kleenex. When my first period surprised me on one of our weekends at the beach, she bought me a package of pads and a soft-serve ice-cream cone at the village convenience store, trying to cheer me up. *It's a pain,* she acknowledged, *but I've had my period your whole life, and have you ever noticed, even once? You throw some Kotex in your bag and go on with your life.*

I found an unopened package of pads in the hall closet and gave it to her. We stood looking at each other, both of us thinking the same thing. Unexplained bleeding was the symptom that had led to her diagnosis the year before. But she'd had two clear scans since finishing treatment. They had told her that she was cancer-free.

"You should call your doctor," I said.

A week later, she was back home in Oregon, undergoing more tests. My husband and kids and I drove to a lakeside cabin in the Adirondacks, where we had planned to end our summer. As beautiful as it was there, I couldn't stop worrying about my mom. I texted her daily, tried calling between dips in the lake and board games with the kids, but she didn't answer.

Finally, on our last night, as we were packing up to leave, she replied to one of my texts. *Sorry I missed your calls. I'm doing okay. Glad you're having fun at the lake! We can talk when you get home.*

That was when I knew that her cancer was back.

14

OF COURSE SHE WANTED TO HEAR ALL ABOUT OUR TRIP first. The pictures looked so pretty. Did the girls like the cabin? Did they swim every day? How was the weather upstate?

Pacing in my bedroom, wearing the sweaty, rumpled clothes I'd traveled home in, I supplied quick, one-word answers, trying not to sound impatient. "Okay," I said at last, gripping my phone tightly, "please tell me what's going on with you. Did you get your test results?"

"Well—" Her voice wavered, and my heart plunged. "I'm afraid it's not good news."

I braced one hand against the wall and waited. Distantly, as if the thought had been formed in someone else's mind before coming to rest in mine: *There can't be* much *cancer. It should be treatable. She had a clean scan a few months ago.* So why did I feel as if I were falling, tumbling through empty air, with nowhere to land?

I heard her say that there was a new growth, larger than the one before, in her abdomen. There was another tumor in her spine, and "spots" in her liver and lungs that were likely new lesions. She didn't say the words *terminal* or *stage 4*. She didn't have to. Still, my mind struggled against the truth.

"What does this mean?" I asked, almost pleading. "I'm sorry, but can you tell me what this means?"

She said, "I think it means I'm going to die," and then she began to cry.

A memory came to me: I was a child, eight or nine, lying awake in my room while a babysitter watched television in our living room. I wasn't in my bed, but curled up in a roll of blankets on the carpet, because at that age I would often lie on the floor when I was too anxious to sleep; there was something about that firmness and resistance, the feeling of all my limbs, my entire small frame, pressing into solid ground, that made me feel safer. No matter how late the hour, I could never fall asleep until my parents got home. *What if they lost control of their car in the rain?* I used to wonder, on those sleepless nights when I waited to hear their car in the driveway, their voices in the hall. *What if they're lying in a ditch right now? What will I do without them? Who will take care of me?*

Neither of us expected fairness in life, especially after Dad's death. But this—this was merciless.

Sitting on the woven rug in my bedroom, warm phone pressed to my ear, I heard myself say a word I had never before said in my mother's presence through sobs that made it hard to breathe. Had I just made her tell me that she was dying? *I shouldn't have asked. I shouldn't have made her say the words.* I hadn't known it was possible to feel so frantic and so utterly empty, panic clanging in a hollow bell. I tried to think of something, anything to say that might be a comfort—I heard myself making pointless promises, saying that she should call me anytime she wanted; that Dan and I would help; that we loved her and would do whatever we could. *I won't be useless to you the way I was to Dad*, I thought.

After she had hung up, I huddled on the floor, pressing my palm to the ache that had bloomed deep in my chest. That was where Dan found me a few moments later. From the anguished look on his face, I could tell that he knew what my mother had told me—our house isn't large, and wails travel easily through the vents. I didn't ask him if our kids had heard me crying. I didn't ask if they were worried. The only child I could think about was me.

He gathered me close and said, *I'm so sorry*, as I sobbed, over and over, *I'm going to lose her. I'm going to lose them both.*

I had not stopped speaking of *my parents* as a collective unit, in the present tense, as if Dad were alive. It still felt wrong to see my mother without him; when she visited, I couldn't stop looking around, wondering where he was. Neither she nor I had learned to live without him yet, though in our own ways, we were trying.

But his death had been the long-feared absence, and so it was, to some degree, the expected one. My mother was the one who survived, the one who was supposed to stay with me for decades to come. I had believed that she would eventually find some measure of peace—that she would get sunburned in Greece, laugh and spend time with her friends from church, see my hair go gray and my kids grow up. It was the life she wanted, the life she deserved. Hers was the loss I never saw coming.

15

IT'S LATE MORNING, THE FOG BURNING OFF TO LET THE green hills peek through, and I'm walking my mother's dog, Buster, up one side of each narrow street, down the other, past row after row of homes. Each little street that branches off from the main road through the mobile-home park is a dead end, and we follow each one to its terminus and back, which means that we have a chance to see every house, every car, every lawn ornament twice per walk. Our circuit through the park takes us fifteen minutes, moving as briskly as Buster's short little legs will allow.

As we near my mother's house, I turn left and walk fifty or so paces to the wood-and-chicken-wire fence you can glimpse from her living room window, one of several separating her neighborhood from nearby farmland. I like to stop and linger here to see the mountains, if they're out. There used to be another draw, a pair of horses that grazed in the tall grass beyond the fence, and I suspect that Buster would bark at the ponies if they were still here. His growls and yippy barks can be unpredictable. But he is the beloved pet of my mother's widowhood, and we've gotten used to each other.

Mom had been anxious about having a pet in Dad's later years—she worried he would trip over a dog or cat, unsteady as he could be on his feet—but if it were only up to her, I knew she would always have a dog in the house. After Dad died, I asked her, *Why not get another dog?*—thinking of the pets we'd had when I was a child, and all the dogs of Mom's girlhood that she had told me stories of: Prince, Stinky, Jughead. I was surprised when she shrugged and said something about dogs needing a lot of time and attention. *I have enough to worry about as it is.* But sure enough, a few months later, I got a picture of her holding a little black dog who looked very pleased to be in her arms. I had to laugh when she told me his name: *buster* has always been my mom's go-to moniker for any young, mischievous male child, related to her or not (she calls girls of the same type *young lady*).

Buster the dog, as I've learned in our brief acquaintance, might as well be her child; he is spoiled and completely devoted to her. Making his dinner is a several-step process that both my husband and I learned with my mother criticizing us at every step. "Dan, would you consider that a *heaping* scoop?" "He can't eat it *dry*, you need to add some hot water so it makes a kind of gravy, and where are the meat scraps I saved to put on top?" Before my mother leaves the house, she turns on the television—always PBS—in the hopes that he will find the voices comforting and feel less lonely. ("Why PBS?" I asked her. "Well, I figure it's at least semi-educational.") I have sometimes wondered if Buster knows how sick she is, if his sharp little nose sniffed out the truth about the cancer that's killing her—since she became ill, she told me, he has shadowed her more closely, sleeping in her bed at night, keeping watch over her. She frets over what will happen to him, though she isn't ready to talk about where he might live when she's gone. *If I'd known this would happen, I wouldn't have gotten him*. For now, all I can tell her is that we will make sure her dog is all right.

Mom hasn't been able to walk Buster for weeks, and I'm sure he misses going out and around the park with her. When I walk him, he does his business with grudging efficiency. I haven't had a dog since childhood and am unused to planning my day around the needs of one. No matter how difficult the day is or how much I want to talk with my mom, everything must stop, three times a day, so that Buster can have his walk. But I'm glad to have a reason to get out and move, to breathe cold, fresh air, to look at something beyond the walls of my mother's house. The pavement is wet from this morning's shower, and Buster and I take detours around the biggest puddles.

The mountains are at once immense and homely, and seem so close I can almost imagine running right into them if we could cross the neighboring field. When I lived here, I used to walk to another field near our old house to watch the sky darken above gold-limned hills. Sometimes, driving home in the evening, I'd pull over to admire the view— the riotous colors of sunset, the slow-deepening blue of the mountains as the light receded. I've relaxed at peaceful eastern lakes and walked along Atlantic beaches, but have yet to find any substitute for these mountains. There's a reason my mother still sends me cards featuring photographs and watercolors of snow-covered peaks and foothills clustered with evergreens—she knows how much I miss the geography of home. Every time I return, it's the Cascades that greet me first, from the window of a small plane. Without words, without answers, they offer me the same peace they always have.

I will lift up mine eyes unto the hills, from whence cometh my help.

I can feel my mind ease a fraction, though my anxieties are slower to dissipate than the strands of fog clinging to the base of the hills. Other than my family, there's little I miss, feel genuinely nostalgic for, in this sheltered valley. But the way I love these mountains, high and stark amid cloud cover and sun-shot sky, is as simple as the comfort of a dog, the promise of an Oregon rain shower. No matter my state of mind when I return, the friendly ranges encircle and welcome me, rising above green and gold fields, too vast to be outgrown; more than anything else, they make me feel that I might still have a place here.

My dad loved this view. I can picture him sitting outside on my parents' patio, wearing a baseball cap and his favorite blue Hawaiian shirt, listening to the radio and watching the hills emerge from the clouds. The day we buried him, there was a sun shower, and we gathered outside to see a rainbow arching over the peaks. Some hours later, when the overcast sky gave way to a fiery orange-and-rose sunset, one of the best I could ever remember seeing, Mom sighed and squeezed my hand. *Quite a send-off.*

My father never feels closer or farther away than when I return to this place to find him gone. Now I'm walking a dog he never met, wondering if he knows what my mother is facing; what we are going through without him. I turn around, the mountains a reassuring wall at my back, and let Buster lead us home for lunch.

16

ON THE DAY AFTER CHRISTMAS, I TOOK MY MOTHER OUT
to her favorite diner.

My husband, kids, and I had flown to Oregon to spend
the week with her, and my sister, Cindy, and her family made
the trip down from Portland with a carful of Christmas decorations to deck the halls of our Airbnb. My mom didn't have
extra beds or space for guests, and we wanted her to be able to
retreat to her own space and have privacy when she needed,
so we had rented a house not far from hers. I drove over each
morning to pick her up and bring her to the Airbnb and drove
her back when she was ready to go to bed. That morning, I'd
thrown on some clothes and stopped for doughnuts on the
way to her place.

While she dug into the sticky pink box, searching for a
maple bar, I tidied up her living room and took Buster out
to do his business. Mom had slipped and fractured her
knee two days before our arrival; she was waiting to see an
orthopedic surgeon, making do with a knee brace and a cane.

We didn't yet know that the break was the result of the cancer eating away at her tibia and femur, or that it would prove unmendable—as the surgeon would put it, *There's not enough healthy bone left to repair.* We didn't know that she would never walk unassisted again. We wouldn't get her latest scan results until after New Year's, and so we were still able to tell ourselves that we might get what her oncologist called *more quality time*—a phrase implying that the quality of her time would slowly leech away as her cancer advanced, until it no longer made sense to continue treatment.

After I unhooked Buster's leash and washed my hands at the kitchen sink, I asked Mom what she wanted for lunch. She thought for a moment, then named her wish: a Reuben sandwich from the diner one town over. We set off in the rental car, and I found myself wishing we had farther to go. It was an afternoon of cold, sunlit beauty in the mountains. I was still struggling to put myself back together after falling apart the night before.

We all had a surprisingly good Christmas together, with a full house of family and friends. My brother-in-law deepfried a turkey. My kids had gotten a mini Polaroid camera for Christmas, and the coffee table soon filled up with their tiny developing portraits. My mother, a largely stationary and therefore easy subject, materialized in shot after shot, sitting on a stranger's couch in her festive burgundy tunic and a necklace of Christmas bells. She was smiling in every picture and clearly having a wonderful time, despite the pain in her knee. I tried to pretend that this was just another holiday, telling myself that I should be happy to be spending it with both my sister and my mother.

Then my husband threw up, and though he told me he thought it was only a delayed travel reaction, or something he'd eaten that disagreed with him, I began to fret about all of us catching a stomach bug and giving it to my immunocompromised mom. My children were more interested in playing with their cousin than they were in visiting with any of the adults, and chafed at our request that they spend more time playing in the living room, where my mother could watch them and enjoy their company. I felt irrationally betrayed by everyone, abandoned to face my worry and heartbreak alone—didn't they understand how important this Christmas was? It might be my last one with my mother, which meant that it had to be perfect, which meant that it could not possibly be good enough.

I held it together as I drove my mother home and returned to the house, but I was close to tears by the time we finished cleaning up and putting the kids to bed. The rage and helplessness I felt had no focus—it was not the fault of a single person—but that didn't stop me from picking a petty argument with Dan. When he refused to give me the spirited fight I wanted, I grabbed the keys to the rental car.

My brother-in-law, who I ran into in the hallway, held out his hands and spoke gently, as if trying not to spook a wild animal. "Where are you going?" he asked me.

"I don't know. I just can't stay here anymore."

"Okay. That's okay. Let one of us come with you."

I should have been grateful, seen the offer for the kindness it was. Instead I told him to get out of my way.

I hadn't even buckled my seat belt when I saw worried texts from Dan and Cindy. I couldn't think of anything to say. Driving around in the frigid dark with no one to yell at, my fury burned itself out, leaving me empty of everything but grief. I soon got lost, as if these weren't the very same roads I'd learned to drive on. Streetlights around me blurred; I couldn't see where I was going.

If my mother is going to die, there's no reason why I shouldn't die, too.

I'd been free from such thoughts for more than a year. Now, hearing the whisper again, I recognized it as a lie, something my mind seized at only because I wanted my own pain to end. I pulled in to the parking lot of a grocery store and texted my friend Jasmine, whom I felt I could talk to because she wasn't here, watching me break down in real time. She was awake——or maybe I'd woken her——and said that I should call her. I don't know how long we talked. Until I had stopped crying. I wiped my eyes and nose with a knit scarf because I had no tissues, and turned the car around.

It took me a while to find my way home. Everyone else was asleep when I crept in, and I was relieved that I wouldn't need to face them yet. I crawled into bed and slept for a few hours before waking to the sound of Dan, Cindy, and Rick helping the kids get breakfast. I got dressed, found the car keys, and snuck out the back door without a word to anyone——which, I supposed, I could add to the growing list of things I would need to apologize for.

I was too ashamed to tell my mother about my outburst, or that I had come to see her on my own this morning because I wanted her to do something for me; I couldn't have said what. She was my mom, and I felt sure that she was the one who'd fix all of this, somehow.

At the diner, we chose a table under a row of vivid abstract landscapes painted by the owner, as usual drawing a few curious glances from patrons who hadn't been expecting to see an older redheaded white woman with her Asian daughter. Mom got the Reuben she'd told me she wanted, and I ordered a hearty farmer's breakfast that made me think of the occasional weekends when my dad would bring me along to the diner where his football pool met. I'd read the Sunday comics and savor my bacon and hash browns while the men, all dads I knew, dissected the week's games, and afterward I would unstick myself from the Naugahyde bench and my father and I would go to a nearby park. It was always special to have a little time alone with him on the weekend, because he had so few of them off.

Sitting in my mother's favorite diner, a warm, well-lit space filled with chairs and tables painted in a cozy kaleidoscope of colors, I struggled to recall the last time we'd gone out to eat together, just the two of us. Mom and I had never really gotten into having "girls' days" together, shopping sprees or spa visits without Dan or my dad or the kids. Those things weren't necessarily her idea of fun, and when we did get to see each other, which wasn't nearly often enough, she wanted to spend time together as a family. Soon, I knew, we would head back to the Airbnb, and her attention would be on the kids. She asked me if they had any big plans for the day. A gingerbread-house-making party, I told her.

Though it was the last thing either of us wanted to talk about, I wondered if I should seize this moment of privacy to once again broach the subject of Mom's advance directives— she had no living will, and had thus far been resistant to discussing anything that had to do with her last wishes. I had printed the necessary forms and brought them along on this trip, hoping that I could get her to fill them out and have them witnessed. They were sitting in the bag I'd looped over my chair.

I couldn't bring myself to mention them.

When we both had only an inch or two of coffee left in our mugs, she brought up Dad. "I wish he were here," she said. "Sometimes I wonder what he would say. It's so hard going through all of this without him."

I had not considered my father an especially calm or steadying influence. When I was in high school and my mother got sick, I knew I couldn't talk to Dad about it; he seemed even more fearful and agitated than I was. When he tried to teach me to drive, he made it as far as our neighbor's mailbox before saying, *I can't do this, turn around*, and never got into a car with me in the driver's seat again. His temper could be unpredictable. He was not what I'd call good in a crisis.

At times, though, he surprised me. I remembered his serene pride at my wedding, the only one of four parents who didn't make me cry or lose sleep that week, and how much it helped to talk to him when I was homesick in my first semester of college. *Tell me all about it, you know my hugs cure the blues.* He was not my idea of a rock, but he was my mother's constant. Her life, for nearly forty-five years. She shouldn't have to fight for her survival without him.

The bright colors in the paintings all around us blurred together. Blinking back tears, I did what I thought Dad would have if he were here: I tried to make her laugh. "You know, it's not like he would have been much help."

I was rewarded with a faint chuckle. "That's probably true. God, he'd be *so* upset."

"He'd be furious. Because this is *bullshit*, Mom," I said.

"I miss him terribly, and sometimes I still can't believe he's gone," she told me. "A part of me—the part that was his wife for forty years—just wants to be with him."

I understood what she was saying. She had thought about halting her treatment.

I knew that as long as there was any hope of gaining more time, she would seize it with both hands. In the months to come, she would fight with a fierceness that would surprise even me. I would watch her struggle and rail against her loss of mobility, independence, the ability to make hard decisions or follow complex conversations, and sometimes I would find myself thinking back to this moment in the diner, the only time she ever admitted to me that she had considered her death without dread. She believed that she would see my father again, and as much as she wanted to live, she longed for that meeting.

"I still feel like I'm married to him, even now," she said. "When you're with someone for that long, you know, you'll always have that life together, even when one of you is gone."

We had just celebrated our second Christmas without my dad. Sometimes, sitting with my mom in the house they'd shared, it was so easy to believe that he was out for a walk, or in another room; that any moment, he would enter and tease one of us, pick an argument, turn on one of his ball games. I knew I'd never get used to seeing her without him. But sometimes she managed to bring him near again.

She was the bridge between us, remembering things even I forgot. When she was gone, would it be like losing him again, too?

We both began to cry, drawing more glances I didn't care about. For a moment, I considered asking her for the reassurance I still craved, a kind of secondhand absolution: Had Dad understood why I lived so far away? Had he understood why it was hard to visit? Had he truly forgiven me before he died? But the weight of these questions felt like too much to lay on her shoulders now. And what if the answer, to any or all of them, was *no*?

Sitting in my mother's favorite diner in a pool of bright winter sunlight, I clung to her hand and kept silent, holding on to the family we had been and still were. We wiped our tears—Mom never went anywhere without tissues in her purse—and tried to talk of the holiday and my daughter's upcoming birthday as we drank our coffee down to the dregs. The papers would sit in my bag for one more day, I decided.

I told myself that I was glad for her unshakable faith, the faith that told her she would see my father again. But I wasn't ready for her to go be with him.

—

Two days later, we stood under heavy rain clouds in the town cemetery. It had poured that morning and would do so again the next day, and I worried that my mother would slip in the mud, but she had a new cane and many sturdy arms to lean on: Dan and me, my sister and brother-in-law, and three of my parents' church friends. "I asked them to be here," Mom said to me in a whisper. "It will give me something to focus on so I don't cry."

My father's new headstone was light enough for us to lift and place in the trunk of our rental car when we picked it up from the engraver's two days after Christmas. Now Dan carefully carried it to my father's grave site, all of us trailing behind. When my mother and her friends had finished praying, I automatically crossed myself the Roman way, left to right, and they bowed and crossed themselves right to left. A cemetery volunteer, Owen, stood at a respectful distance, waiting for us to clear out so he could secure the headstone in a base of freshly poured cement.

The cemetery, wreathed in tall oaks, firs, and pines, dated back to pioneer days; now, Owen had told me, he and his wife and a few other volunteers ran the place. I walked over to introduce myself and thank him for his help, handing over a check to pay for the plot next to my father's. His eyes were warm as he shook my hand and gave me a blue folder containing my receipt and a map of the cemetery, the new plot marked with yellow highlighter.

"Hopefully you won't need this for a good long time," he said. "But it'll be here when you do." My eyes filled, not because of his words so much as how he said them, blending professional duty with easy kindness.

When I returned to where my family stood, it took conscious effort not to stare at the empty space to the left of Dad's plot. Mom put her arm around my shoulders, and for a moment I forgot that I was the one who was supposed to be supporting her. "It's beautiful, hon," she said, her voice muffled in my hair. "Thank you for taking care of this for Dad. I don't think I could have done it."

I nodded, not because I thought she ought to thank me, but because I knew that she was right—for reasons I still didn't understand, marking my father's grave was the one thing she hadn't been able to do for him. For months after he died, all she would say was that she would get around to it eventually. "I know this is really important to you," she would acknowledge whenever I brought it up, her tone one of resignation and bewilderment, as if she just could not believe I cared so much about whether Dad ever got a headstone. When your mother is dying, you try to avoid unnecessary arguments—a tough assignment, in my case—but one day I couldn't stop myself from saying, "I didn't *invent* the tradition of marking graves, Mom."

Then her cancer returned with a vengeance, and she told me that when the time came, she wanted to be buried next to Dad. She'd been unable to resist a morbid joke. "If you wait long enough, maybe you can get one headstone for both of us!"

I spoke with the engraver she had found months ago but never called. An artist of few words, he emailed me photographs of the slabs he had available—unpolished rectangles of blue-gray slate that all looked much the same to my undiscerning eye—and told me to go ahead and pick one. I could see why my mother liked the look of these natural stones: they were rustic, a little rough but somehow lovely, too, and well suited to my dad, who used to love hunting for interesting river rocks and knotty twists of driftwood to bring home and arrange in his garden or hosta bed. After Mom chose her favorite, I passed along some text for the engraving, keeping it simple: Dad's full name, his birth and death dates, and a line from the Paschal Troparion my mother had asked her friends to sing at his burial, though he had died in midwinter.

Standing beside his grave, admiring the newly placed headstone, she told me she had chosen this plot for him because we could see the town high school across the street from where we stood. "There are always people coming and going over there, so I knew he wouldn't be lonely," she said, then added with a grin: "And he can hear the football games every Friday!" This was so ridiculous that I had to laugh, which of course was her intention. I liked it when she joked about him, spoke of him in the present tense. Our lives may be linear, finite, but our love for each other is not so easily confined.

"Dad would have loved his headstone," she told me. Again, I agreed. But what mattered most to me was that *she* liked it, that it was what she wanted for him. That, in the end, she had allowed me to do this one needful thing.

17

MY MOTHER'S LIVING ROOM WAS DARK. THOUGH IT WAS only 2:00 p.m. Storm clouds had been hanging over the valley since my arrival the night before. As I went to turn on more lights, I heard her say, "This is all happening so fast."

Her friend Paula looked up from her steno pad. *Consider me your hands and feet in Oregon,* she had told me. For the last two hours, she had been taking notes, creating lists of calls to make, emails to send, banks to visit, forms to have witnessed and notarized. The next day, she would type everything up in a spreadsheet and send it to me: *I've listed all the to-do items in black and added progress notes in green. Feel free to choose a color and add your own notes.* She reached over to touch my mother's hand, offering her a reassuring smile.

"We know it's hard," she said. "That's why we're here to help you."

Elizabeth, another friend from my mother's church, nodded and leaned forward in her chair. "Remember, you're not alone. We're all with you."

"And think of what a good, loving daughter you have," Paula added.

I heard myself laugh, but there was little humor in it. "She'll be ready to give me back after today," I said.

No one else chuckled. Paula and Elizabeth said, "No!" in unison. Mom only shook her head. *I was joking*, I wanted to say to her. *Like you were when I was five or six and got so mad at you that I said I was going to find "my real mom"—remember, you pointed and said, "There's the door"?*

Now that I thought about it, I wondered if she had been joking.

I couldn't believe that our Christmas visit was only a few weeks ago. Since then, the entire landscape of her illness had shifted, and the faint hope we'd once possessed seemed distant now, lost beyond uncrossable miles.

———

A few days after returning home from Oregon, Dan and I hosted his parents and sister for a belated second Christmas. We were opening the last few presents when my mother called and told me that a friend from church was driving her to the emergency room.

"I just woke up on the floor, unconscious," she said. "I think I must have had a seizure."

At the hospital, scans revealed that the round of chemotherapy she'd completed right before Christmas had no effect on her fast-growing cancer. As bad as this was, it paled beside the news that the seizure had been caused by metastasis to her brain. I booked flights back to Oregon and spent all the next day on the phone with specialists who shared conflicting opinions about the available treatments and social workers who described potential home health-care arrangements that neither my mother nor I (nor, so far as I could see, anyone but a billionaire) could afford. All of them assumed that, as her next of kin, I would be the one discussing her options with her. I was tempted to tell them that they were talking to the wrong person; I couldn't even get her to write a will.

What do I have to leave to anyone? she'd asked me once.

"Of course you know that your mother is a very strong and stubborn woman," one of her doctors said to me. "That's partly how she's made it this far."

I filled a dozen sheets of notebook paper with names and phone numbers, questions and explanations and bulleted lists, and then tried to provide the simplest, most digestible synopsis for my mother. The truth neither of us wanted to admit aloud was that, in the wake of her seizure, she was having trouble holding on to what the doctors or I said to her, sometimes forgetting the details after we spoke. She was exhausted and understandably overwhelmed by the glut of information, anxious and still recovering in her hospital room, *making plans one day at a time*, as she told me. Half of our conversations ended with her saying she couldn't talk about this now; we would have to talk about it later.

But there were decisions that couldn't wait many more days, because the brain tumor—which her doctors believed was fast growing—had completely changed the terrain and timeline of her disease. After I had a chance to question three different oncologists over seven hours, their combined thoughts boiled down to two treatment options: she could undergo radiation to shrink the brain tumor, or have surgery to remove it. None of them recommended further chemotherapy or treatment of the primary tumors, the metastasis we had already known about. The brain tumor, they said, demanded our immediate attention, because it had started a countdown.

The final option was no treatment at all, but hospice care. The hospice intake nurse I spoke to was kind but candid. "Whatever your mother decides about treatment, *now* is the time to be making arrangements," she told me. "You need to be able to pay her bills once she can't, so she keeps her house and her lights stay on. She will need you or someone else to make important decisions when she is no longer able to. And if she decides not to treat the brain tumor at all, you should know that you're probably looking at weeks."

I did not know how to ask the question. "Weeks before . . . ?"

"Weeks before your mother is no longer the person you know," she said, more gently.

Mom was firmly opposed to a brain resection after meeting with the surgeon, who'd spent less than five minutes with her and told her she should have the operation if she wanted to live. Brain surgery at this stage felt like too extreme and risky an option to her—how much time could it possibly buy her, even if the brain tumor was successfully removed, when she had inoperable tumors in her pelvic cavity, her bones, her lungs, her liver? She also felt uncertain about the less aggressive treatment, targeted brain radiation; she worried that she would suffer cognitively or lose her memory. But when I talked to the radiation oncologist, who was by far the most patient and compassionate doctor I spoke with that week, he said that he hoped my mother would consider one week of brain radiation sessions in his lab. He felt there was minimal risk to her brain function and assured me that it was absolutely not a desperate attempt to prolong her life at any cost.

"At this point, I wouldn't recommend *any* treatment if it was just about buying her a little more time." As painful as this was to hear, I appreciated his frankness. "This is really about the quality of the time she has left. She's at very high risk of having another seizure or a stroke if the brain tumor is allowed to keep growing. I'm not sure she really understands that most patients with untreated brain tumors eventually kind of . . . drift away."

"What does that mean?"

A brief silence followed, not long enough for me to fill with all my wild guesses. "If she does nothing to treat it, the most typical scenario would mean she would become detached from reality, stop talking, stop eating, stop being aware of loved ones," he said. "She would most likely become comatose before she died. I can't tell you how long she would have—no one can tell you that; every case is different—but I imagine it would be a matter of weeks, maybe a month or two at most, depending on how fast the brain tumor is growing."

I could imagine none of this. "I understand that she has to decide, soon, one way or the other. But I don't think she's quite sure how to do that," I told him.

"Your mother still has the ability and the right to make these choices for herself, but she's recovering from a seizure and is already affected by the brain tumor. That will get worse, and quickly, if it's not treated at all." I could tell that he chose every word carefully. For all his gentleness, his tone brooked no argument. "Even with treatment, this cancer is going to end her life. Some might say that dying from brain cancer is an easier way to go than others, because usually it isn't very painful. Whereas if she tries the brain radiation treatments, that could slow or even stop the growth of the tumor and give her more time as herself. It all depends on what she wants."

We were so far beyond anything my mother might have wanted. I pressed the now-omnipresent ache in my chest, my palm moving in a slow circle over my heart as I tried to breathe and focus on the question directly before us. *This first. Then you can fall apart.*

I was leaving for Oregon the next day, but I also knew that every day might make a difference, so I called my mother to tell her what I'd learned. In my memory, it is more like a conversation I overheard than one I participated in—I felt as though I had stepped outside my own body, heard my voice as if it were a stranger's. I only managed to keep my voice calm because I knew how important it was for her to grasp the stakes.

I explained that without any treatment at all, she could soon lose her awareness, her consciousness, her tether to the people she loved. This was the last major decision she would need to make about her treatment, and she was the only one who could make it. "I don't want to pressure you into getting radiation," I said. "I know you don't want to have brain surgery, and I totally understand and agree with that. If you decide you're all done with treatments and you're ready to enter hospice now, I promise I will support you in that, too. I just want you to understand the choice you're making, and what it means if you *don't* have radiation to treat the brain tumor."

I don't know how either of us made it through that call. Every word had to fight its way out of me. I didn't want to be the one telling her this. I didn't want any of it to be true.

When I said that she would get to a point where she might not know anyone, I felt something shift in the quiet between us. The radiation oncologist hadn't told her any of this, she said, after a long pause. I knew that he had tried. She told me that she would call him. I waited until the oncologist let me know that he had spoken with her again, and then I called her back.

"He said that I should discuss it with you this weekend, and give him my decision on Monday." Her laugh was brittle. "Did you tell him to say that?"

"I don't tell your doctors what to say to you," I said, stung.

"Well, he seemed to think I needed to talk to you to fig- ure out what to do, and I thought that was funny. As though I'm not capable of making decisions without consulting you."

I knew that she was in pain, in shock, and desperately afraid. I told myself that any resentment she might feel toward me was bound to be short-lived; she loved me with her whole being; she wouldn't push me away now, right when I felt the urge to cling to her. But I'd been living with my own grief and terror for months, and we had so little time. She was the only parent I had left. I *knew* that she needed me now, whether she wanted to admit it or not——I needed her to trust me, let me help her, let me be her daughter.

"Why wouldn't you talk about this decision with me?" I said, my voice cracking. "I'm your only child. It would be a normal thing to do. Who would you rather talk to about it?"

"Oh, for heaven's sake," she bit off, "calm down. I can't handle you getting hysterical on me. We'll talk about it when you come home."

She hung up.

I stood alone in my kitchen, fingers itching to hurl my phone against the wall. If she was going to accuse me of hysteria, shouldn't I at least get to *be* hysterical—to scream and sob, watch fragile objects shatter? Before I could do more than eye my water glass, imagine the satisfying crash of it hitting the cold tile, I heard my husband's voice upstairs. One of my daughters responded, words I couldn't make out, and giggled.

This was no time, no place for me to break down. I tried to redirect my thoughts, focus my flagging energy on what had to be done. My mother needed to make a decision about radiation. She needed to write a will. And, as the hospice intake nurse had explained, she needed to empower me or someone else to pay her bills and apply for any assistance she might require once she was unable to do so herself.

My mind churned, pushing past my rising panic, and a name rose to the surface: Elizabeth. The person my mother had chosen to make health-care decisions if she couldn't, whose name was listed on the forms she had finally filled out at Christmas, whose number was now stored in my phone for this reason. Mom had wanted someone local, who could quickly get to the hospital and have eyes on the situation, and I could see at once why she had chosen Elizabeth, a calm and compassionate friend from church who worked in the medical field and was familiar with loss. Surely it wouldn't be a betrayal, I thought, to call and ask her for advice? This was my mother's medical power of attorney, after all. She might be called on to exercise that responsibility sooner rather than later.

I sent a hesitant text and Elizabeth responded at once, inviting me to call her. We spoke for more than an hour. As we talked, I felt my heart rate gradually slow, the pain in my chest ease. She agreed that my mother was overwhelmed, for good reason, and had to make some big decisions, but suggested that perhaps she needed to hear all of this from someone who wasn't her child.

"No matter how old you get, you're still our kids, and we want to protect you," she told me. "Now, you're coming out tomorrow, you said. Do you want me to be there with you when you talk with your mom?"

That was exactly what I wanted, though I hadn't realized it until she made the suggestion. Elizabeth said that she would come over on Saturday afternoon, and she would ask their friend Paula to be there as well. "Paula is the most organized person I know," she said. "She loves your mom, and I know she'll want to help." I thanked her and went to pack for the trip, grateful once again for my mother's stalwart friends.

———

Elizabeth had been right: my mother needed to talk with someone who wasn't me. When her friends asked what she wanted to do with her home, she immediately said that her sister, who was moving in to help her, should inherit it. What about the car? She was no longer able to drive, and had decided to donate her car to the church. The money from her small life insurance policy should be split between my children, she told us. She wasn't ready to discuss funeral arrangements, but we knew which rites and services she wanted, and Paula shared the name and phone number of a funeral home that had been recommended by their priest.

Together, we filled out the simplest will and financial power of attorney forms my husband had been able to find online. Mom agreed to add me to her bank accounts so that I could pay her bills and transfer money from my own account if needed. Finally, we turned to the looming question of radiation. It was clear that she had been thinking about everything the radiation oncologist had told her. As her designated health-care agent, Elizabeth began with gentle, probing questions, and Mom ultimately decided she would try the recommended treatment. It wouldn't be a cure, nor was it meant to be, but hopefully it would slow the brain tumor's growth and help ensure that she stayed *with* us for as long as she was with us. Then she would begin hospice care.

Before they left, Elizabeth and Paula each took one of my mother's hands. "Forgive me any offenses, my sister," they said, one after the other.

My mother said, "I forgive you, and God forgives you."

I hadn't observed anything that afternoon that I thought anyone should feel sorry for, but the three friends seemed to take comfort in the ritual. All accepted the simple exchange of forgiveness as a matter of fact—in a communion of smiles, a squeeze of the hand, and friendly words that took on the weight of a prayer, any small, overlooked fractures in their relationships were wholly restored. I was so moved that it took me a few moments to recognize the other emotion twisting through my heart: I was envious. While her friends got to ask her for forgiveness and start afresh at every meeting, this seemed much harder for a grown daughter to do.

I walked Paula and Elizabeth to the door and thanked them for their help. They hugged me, whispered some encouragement, and drove away in their separate cars, windshield wipers on in the late-afternoon drizzle. Back inside, I asked Mom if I could get anything for her, and she shook her head. She looked exhausted. Of course she was, after what we'd put her through the last two hours.

Earlier in the day, my eleven-year-old had disappeared into the spare room, headphones on, to watch a movie on her tablet while the adults talked. I had brought her with me because I knew she wouldn't get many more visits with her grandma, and also because when she begged to come along, I was relieved to think that I'd have her for company, her sweet and steady presence another reason for me to keep it together. She looked more like me the older she got, but she was her father's child. Somewhere between my dad's death and my mom's illness, she'd grown up so much, become another person I could rely on, though sometimes I felt guilty for doing so.

I knocked on the door, opened it to tell her that we were done. "Thank you for being so patient," I said. "I think Grandma would really love your company right now."

She nodded, already getting to her feet. "Did her friends help you? Did you get all your forms filled out?"

My forms. That was how my mother thought of them, too. I was grateful to know that so many choices and contingencies were discussed and settled, recorded in black and white, and ready to be witnessed. I wouldn't have been able to forgive myself had I not tried to explain the reality of her situation and her treatment options, helped her take steps to ensure that she could remain secure in her home for as long as she wanted, asked her to voice her final wishes while she still could. Yet I felt precious little relief, now that the job was done.

I had been living beyond my parents' help or easy reach for more than half my life. I had learned how to take care of myself; since I was sixteen, I had been telling them about my choices, only rarely asking them what I should do. While I had been living independently of them, they had also been living independently of *me*: I was not someone they had regularly consulted when weighing a decision, big or small. They did not rely on me for day-to-day assistance. Even when my mother learned that she was dying, she did not want to uproot what was left of her life and come live with me.

I had thought it my responsibility to try to step into my father's place somehow, even if I had to do so from afar; supporting Mom however she needed, helping her make crucial decisions and live on her own terms for as long as she could, was now my job, wasn't it? But we'd had so little time to figure out our relationship, learn what it would be without my father. In her view, I was a child, her child—an adult, perhaps, but not a peer. It was not possible for me to replace my dad as her adviser, her right hand. She did not think about leaning on or drawing strength from me, but of protecting me, lifting me up. To her, that was what it meant to be my mother.

18

LIFE IS ANYTHING BUT NORMAL WHEN YOUR MOTHER IS dying. I drag the knowledge that I will lose mine through every day, every moment. And yet the first two months of 2020 *are* normal compared with what will follow. There are so many things I can and do take for granted, like my children's health, my family's safety, our daily routines of work and school, my ability to get on a plane and fly anywhere. I travel to Oregon and back again. I attend a conference at the end of February, around the time my mother begins hospice care: I hug colleagues, shake dozens of hands, eat elbow to elbow with strangers in crowded rooms, not knowing that in a few weeks all of this will feel like a fantasy borrowed from another universe.

By March, we can't go an hour without hearing of another emergency cancellation. Businesses, basketball games, book tours, baby showers—every aspect of life, it seems, has been disrupted by COVID-19. The kids' schools close. We're asked to stay home, shelter in place, but when the request comes from overburdened nurses and doctors wearing trash bags instead of the medical-grade PPE they need, it sounds more like a plea. We no longer see anyone outside our immediate household, unless it's over a screen. My best friend one neighborhood away feels almost as far as my sister in Portland. I stress over which key supplies and shelf-stable foods to buy, stock up on my asthma medicine, and try not to touch my face.

I had planned to visit my mother again in mid-March, with a family trip to follow during the kids' spring break in April. There are no more forms to fill out, no more fraught decisions to make; Mom and I just want to spend more time together while we can. The day before my flight, March 13, I call and say that I'm going to postpone my trip. She agrees it's probably for the best. "Hopefully this will be over soon, and you and the kids can fly out in a month or two," she says.

I want my children to have at least one more chance to see their grandma. But with each passing day, it's harder to imagine traveling across the country with them. We know so little about the virus in these early days. Is it airborne? Spread via surfaces? Do cloth masks really help? How badly do kids suffer when they get it? How much risk is compounded if you have coexisting conditions, as I do, or a developmental disability, as my younger daughter does? If one of us picks it up while we're traveling, will we pass it to my immunocompromised mother, or her hospice nurse, or her other caregivers?

At least, I tell myself, Mom's current risk of exposure is about as low as it gets. She lives in a town of a few thousand people, hundreds of miles from the nearest major outbreak. She and her sister, who recently moved in to care for her, have a handful of masked visitors—a few of my mother's friends from church, her hospice nurse, her priest—but Mom never leaves home anymore. While we now know that she won't get better, she has been enjoying a "stable period," according to her nurse. If I travel to see her now, no matter how careful I try to be in the air, or while transferring planes at LAX or SFO or SEA, I could be the one to carry the virus to her and compromise this fragile, hard-won stability.

It also feels as though I'd be abandoning a household in shambles if I left. While Dan and I are both working from home now, as a scientist he is considered essential personnel and expects he'll need to go back in eventually, and it's not easy for either of us to get a full day's work done with schools closed. It gets harder still when remote learning begins in earnest; our kids are grieving, isolated, irritable, and bored, and the last thing they want is to be assigned hours of busywork on a Chromebook. Our younger daughter's Individualized Education Program—all the supports and accommodations we spent years advocating for and hammering out at stressful meetings with her school team—has essentially disappeared overnight. At school, she has a one-to-one aide; at home, she has us: Dan takes the math block, I take language arts, and we split the other subjects. If one of us didn't sit with her for every lesson, she'd be unable to manage the multiple online platforms or access her schoolwork at all.

There are always dozens of tabs open on my phone: flights home, a smaller number every day; articles about virus transmissibility; articles analyzing (guessing at) the risks of flying; tables showing infection rates where I live, and in the cities I might have to fly through, and in my mother's county. One morning, while struggling to pay attention to my daughter's reading-group Zoom lesson, I think about how responsibly attempting a solo trip at this moment would mean two weeks of quarantine at either end, in addition to however long I spent with my mom. I have never left Dan and the kids for that long, not even for my book tour, and it doesn't feel like an option now. Our home life, our jobs, our routines—none of this is set up for one of us to parent alone, for weeks or months, while working remotely and dealing with anxious, homebound children. And what if I somehow gave the virus to my mother? What if I came back and gave it to my family? What if I passed it to someone far more vulnerable, whose name I would never know, whose illness or death I would never be aware of causing?

I can't afford to wallow or be idle while juggling work and virtual school, and yet a part of me remains ever still and watchful, as if I were holding my breath, waiting for something it feels too risky to name. Surely, I think, in quiet moments, we're bound to get a reprieve soon. We will remember our responsibilities to one another. Those who are able to stay home will stay home, everyone will start wearing masks in public spaces, caseloads will drop, and it will feel safe—*safer*—to go see my mom.

Instead, as the weeks go by, mask wearing is politicized, public health experts are frequently ignored, and people who look like me are scapegoated and attacked, accused of causing the pandemic. Hospitals fill as the virus keeps raging.

—

My grandmother's memory-care facility has been locked down for weeks. Grandma went from seeing family several times a week to seeing no one at all, and she is struggling. She stops eating, stops getting out of bed, stops responding to questions. She's put on hospice care in early April and is allowed visitors then, but in her fragile health my mother can't go, nor can she don the full protective gear required. Though they are separated by only a few miles, she will lose her mother sight unseen.

When Grandma dies on April 7, two months shy of ninety-six, we think of her as another casualty of the pandemic. She didn't die of COVID, but she was unable to face the isolation of the nursing home that had locked down early for patients' safety. I remember how she would greet me when I came home—*is this really our Nicole?*—and that she never forgot me, no matter how many memories she lost. Yet I find it's hard to access my grief for her, or rather to disentangle it from my anticipatory grief for my mother. When Mom tells me that she wasn't ready for Grandma to go—*you're never really ready to lose your mother*—I want to tell her that I know.

I ask, tentatively, if I should try to fly out for the burial. "Better not," she says. "There's nothing you could do if you were here. We'll have a funeral for her later, when it's safe."

At this stage of the pandemic, without adequate testing and no idea how widespread infections are, every newly deceased person is treated as if they had COVID and may still be infectious. No one is allowed to view my grandmother's body. No one can be present when she is buried next to Grandpa at the local veterans' cemetery. A few days later, when my mother and her sister go together to lay flowers on their parents' graves, it is the first time my mom has left the house in weeks.

——

Sometimes, it's almost easy to picture driving to Dulles or National or BWI. Walking through the glass doors of the airport with my roller bag. What's much harder to imagine is coming into contact with thousands of people, touching all those common surfaces, breathing all that common air. Getting on a plane, and landing at another airport, and getting on another plane, and landing at a third airport. Along the way, in the twelve, fourteen, sixteen hours it would take me to get home, how many strangers would I meet? How many restrooms would I use? How many times would I have to pull my mask down to eat something, to drink water?

I think about my mother on a ventilator in the hospital, unable to have any visitors. I think about me and my risk factors and the possibility of not being here for my own kids. I imagine one of them in the hospital, struggling to breathe, confused, terrified, alone. And that is always where my mind spins to a stop.

As the days go by and virtual work and learning continue, our children's discontent hardens into bored resignation. I start polling others about what I should do, partly because it is so hard to trust my own sanity and judgment. My questions are always the same, but a few patient friends pick up every single time to listen to me run through the terrible choices. Everyone is quick to say that they wouldn't blame me for going. But they also don't think I should travel across the country, not right now.

"If it were *only* you, and you didn't have kids, and you were close enough to get there on a short, direct flight, I'd say go," my friend Nicole tells me one day. "But you do have kids. A whole day of travel? All those cars and planes, all the people who aren't wearing masks? We don't know enough about how this thing spreads, we don't have any good treatments that can knock it back, and now there's this multisystem inflammatory syndrome some kids are getting."

I'm standing under the dogwood tree in my backyard, where I often take phone calls now—outside, so my kids won't hear me cry. Every tree and plant in sight is blooming, bursting with new life, and it feels like a mockery. It's raining, a light spring drizzle. I estimate that I have about three more minutes to talk on the phone here before I'll need to make a run for it.

"I can't bear this," I say.

"Of course you can't," she says. "It's unbearable. You know that episode of *Star Trek* where Counselor Troi is trying to become a commander?"

Saturday-night *Star Trek* was appointment television for me and my dad, so I know very well that the Troi commander storyline is the B plot in the seventh-season *Star Trek: The Next Generation* episode "Thine Own Self." In it, Troi keeps trying and failing to pass a particular bridge officer's test, which happens to be a test not of technical skill or problem-solving ability but of duty and grit. When she fails, as she does multiple times, it's because she will not accept that which feels impossible to accept. She finally realizes that while she has been trying to save the ship without losing anyone—without sending a friend, a person she serves with and cares for, to die—giving that order is the only way to pass the test. As soon as she tells a holographic crewmate to sacrifice himself for the good of the ship, the simulated disaster ends and she is promoted.

"Your kids, your husband, they are your ship now," Nicole says. "They're your priority. Even though it's the hardest thing, and it's so unfair, because your mother is dying and there's a fucking pandemic and none of this should be happening. You do what you need to do to save the ship."

———

My kids, I find, are what I cannot risk.

Mom is aware that I'm wrestling with the decision of whether to travel. She's torn, because of course she wants us to visit. But she's also been following the news, if not as obsessively as I have. She says she'll understand no matter what I decide.

I'm grateful to know she doesn't blame me for wanting to protect her and my children. But I already know what it is to blame myself for distance, for time missed. For months now, we've gotten nothing but terrible news, but at least until the pandemic we were able to see each other. I thought we would get more visits, more time together—the time I didn't get with Dad. I thought I'd be beside her when she died. Now I don't know if I will ever see her again.

19

***

THINGS I SEND TO MY MOTHER WHILE SHE IS DYING

Letters and cards

Flowers

Watercolor artwork and comics drawn by my kids

A small Christmas tree in a ceramic pot, with decorations

All the good Jane Austen film adaptations I can find on DVD that she doesn't already own

The complete *Slings & Arrows*

The complete *Miss Fisher's Murder Mysteries*

The complete *Poirot*

All the Harriet Vane/Peter Wimsey novels

Most of Helen Mirren's film oeuvre

A new tablet to replace her old one, with Skype preinstalled

An Oregon sunstone necklace

Warm socks

Nice hand lotion

Good coffee

Chicken soup and rolls

Pears

Chocolate babka

Chocolate-chip cookies

Mother's Day tulips

A new knee brace

20

I KNOW, ON DAYS WHEN SHE GETS ANGRY, THAT SHE IS not really angry with me. She is grieving for her mother. She is grieving for herself. Despite her faith in God's mercy, the existence of heaven, the promise of seeing my father again, she wants to live.

She still has some good days, but she has more and more hard ones. One night, she has a fall that leaves her with a bruise on her forehead, and when I call her, she sounds confused and furious. *I don't understand what's wrong with me. I don't know why this is happening.*

Soon, she can't text or write emails anymore. The very last text she sends me, in mid-April, is about her plan to visit my grandmother's grave. The last email is a couple of lines asking what the kids might want for Easter, because she's determined to keep sending them gifts and treats. From then on, we have only phone calls or video calls. But they're not always easy to coordinate, and sometimes she cannot easily follow the conversation; it's the brain tumor, her nurse tells me, as well as the pain medication.

I want her to have something tangible, something she can hold on to, so I write her a letter—on lighthouse stationery, because it makes me think of all the weekends we spent together on the Oregon coast. Beach trips with my grandmother were always busy, packed with crabbing and clamming, shopping and bike rides, fishing in the bay, card games all evening. Trips with my mom were quiet and slow, consisting of long walks by the ocean and greasy diner meals and a visit to our favorite lighthouse, where a hundred-mile-long river flowed into the bay. The lighthouse gift shop was her favorite, which is why I have T-shirts, salt and pepper shakers, place mats, pencils, and refrigerator magnets all adorned with lighthouses. She is probably the one who sent me the stationery.

I fill several sheets of paper, telling her how much we miss her and wish we were with her. I tell her that the kids loved seeing her at Christmas, and that they talk about her all the time. I tell her that she's the one who taught me how to be a parent, how to put my children first. That her love was the foundation of my life, and her belief in me is what made everything I've ever done possible. I tell her how brave she is. After I mail the letter, I ask her friends and caregivers to keep it close at hand and read it to her whenever she asks.

She is well cared for by her sister, who lives nearby and has moved in to help her, and their sister-in-law, who has flown in to assist. At night there are home health aides, whom we're able to pay only because my mother cashed out her small IRA prior to starting hospice care. Less than a year of her income, it would not have been enough for her to live on if she had more time. It might be enough for her to die on.

The invoices the home health-care agency sends me total thousands of dollars per week. My mother's money will soon be gone, but I have a backup plan: the emergency fund that Dan and I have been fortunate to save in the last year, which we have already been using to help support Mom, and a concurrent Medicaid application. Medicare alone won't be nearly enough, I've learned from my research, and Medicaid will likely take weeks to be approved and cover only a portion of the care she needs, but I don't know what else to do except try once the money runs out.

I do my best to keep up with her other bills, stay in touch with her hospice team and the home health-care agency, send her flowers and gifts from afar. I am continually thankful that I'm able to do this for her, though it doesn't feel like enough; I am spared the guilt I felt when I was unable to provide any meaningful assistance to my dad. But I cannot see how anyone is able to pay for home health care for years on end. I do the math and realize how quickly it could bankrupt us all if my mother had longer to live.

———

The days blur together, slip away. Everything has changed. Nothing changes. Here is my bedroom, my office, my kitchen, my yard. Here are emails that need answering, remote school lessons to attend, video meetings to run. Here are long walks with my kids, books I can't focus on, meals I don't feel like eating. Here is another call with Mom.

When I call, I feel as if I need to apologize. I know that I am pestering her caregivers with still more tasks: giving me updates, seeing whether she can speak with me, bringing her the phone or tablet. I feel like a nuisance, not only to them, but to her. Sometimes she holds the tablet herself; other times, she needs someone to do it for her. It's harder and harder for her to carry on a conversation. But I keep calling, afraid to go even one day without at least trying to reach her. I am afraid of the day when I will no longer hear her voice.

On an afternoon when she sounds more cognizant of her situation than she has in many days, we both break down. I tell her that she doesn't deserve any of this. "None of this is fair to you," I say. "You deserve to have your daughter with you."

She tells me that she understands why I'm not there, but I'm not sure if I will ever understand.

When the kids and I call her another day, she is looking more like her old self, perhaps because she's wearing her glasses—nearsighted as she is without them, I've noticed she rarely has them on for our video calls—and one of my father's old Cleveland Browns T-shirts. I can tell that she is weak, and she has lost more weight, though she says that she still eats well. From the sound of her voice, she has recently woken from a nap. She holds up the flowers we sent her and thanks us, but even from the other side of a screen I can see that the online shop I ordered from has failed us. More than half the blooms are wilted.

May rolls around, and toward the end of one particularly long day, I text a friend: *I think Mom forgot my birthday*. It's understandable, I think. It's more and more difficult for her to talk on the phone or over Skype. She's on pain meds that are only available to the dying, the kind of medication she refused when she first started hospice care, and she is sleeping more often. I wouldn't be surprised if she no longer keeps close track of the days.

I'm about to head upstairs to get ready for bed when my phone rings. *Mom* flashes on the screen. My breath catches. When I answer, she doesn't even say hello. We both know why she is calling.

"Happy birthday to you . . ."

She sings with as much life as she can, more than I've heard from her in days. I wonder if I should tell her to save her strength. I know this call is an effort. But I also know that she called because she believes this is important: she's my mother, and she has a job to do.

After I left home, my parents called on every birthday to sing to me—Dad in his gravelly baritone, Mom enthusiastic and slightly off-key—and she has continued the tradition alone since he died. She always sends me a card, too, and sometimes flowers, but the birthday call is the most important part of the long-distance celebration: sacrosanct, for all that I have taken it for granted.

"Happy birthday to you . . ."

After she sings the first two lines, she takes a shuddery

breath and surprises me with an edit. "Your mom didn't forget your birthday, and she really loves you."

Tears are rolling down my face. My husband, sitting next to me on the couch—close enough to have heard my mother singing—reaches over to take my hand, squeezing it hard. All of us know it's the last birthday call. I manage to thank her with only a little wobble in my voice.

"Well, of course," she says. "I just woke up from a nap and thought, I'd better call Nikki. I'm glad I made it in time."

21

THE WEEK AFTER MOTHER'S DAY, HER HOSPICE NURSE
calls me. "She had a great day! She's such a fighter—she has
a real chance at more quality time."

It seems too good to be true, but of course I am desperate
to believe it after so many bleak days. When I get ahold of
Mom, my husband and kids join me in crowding around my
phone. I tell her how glad we are to hear she's had a good day
and that we wish we were with her. She speaks slowly, with
some effort, and sometimes forgets to hold the tablet at the
right angle, so we can see only part of her face. I'm always
afraid now, but after hearing about her afternoon—sitting
up, eating ice cream, even joking with people—I tell myself
that anyone in her condition would be tired after such a full
day. Her nurse said she might have more time, and this is all
I want, so I let myself hope.

"I love you all," she says to us. "Never, never forget how
much I love you."

It's the last time we'll hear her voice.

———

Until the pandemic, I expected that I would be with her at the end. That was the trade-off, I thought. She shouldn't be dying at all, but if she had to die, at least we would know that it was coming. I'd get the call, I'd get on a plane, she would hold on until I arrived. I would hold her hand, and we would get to say goodbye.

Instead, we had calls across time zones, conversations that grew shorter and shorter by the day. Blurry faces on a range of screens. Tears over the phone. Texts I sent long after she stopped replying. And finally, silence, when the calls stopped.

I can't tell you about her death, because I didn't witness it.

———

When I call on Saturday, her sister-in-law texts back to tell me that it's hard for Mom to speak. She's been sleeping all day. I want to talk to her, even if she can't respond, but I decide not to press. I thank her for letting me know and say that I'll try again the next day.

On Sunday morning, I send another text: *If it's possible today, I would just like to tell Mom that we love her.*

Before I go to bed, I text again, reiterating that the next time she is even slightly alert, we'd appreciate it so much if someone would hold the phone up so we can send our love.

When my phone rings on Monday, I still hope to hear a voice telling me that my mother is awake and able to listen. Instead, I hear the words "Your mom is gone."

"No," I say.

"It was peaceful," my aunt says. "It was time, honey. The cancer was everywhere. It was time for her suffering to end."

I want to ask her to tell me more, but what is there to say now? I want to offer some kind of help, but what can I possibly do? I apologize, although I don't know why—maybe because I am crying, heaving too hard to speak—and ask if I can call her later. She says I can call whenever I want.

My entire family is home, because my entire family is always home now. My husband hears me and comes running, my daughters know what has happened before we tell them.

For the rest of the day and most of the night, I cannot stop crying. I cry while I eat or drink. I cry in the shower, and when I lie down to try to sleep. Even when I am worn out, too hoarse for my sobs to make much of a sound, the tears keep coming, silently drifting down my cheeks.

All I can think about is how, at the end, I wasn't with her. She was the kind of mother who deserved to have her child there when she died. Knowing that I had her steadfast support, that she loved and believed in me no matter what, made me so much braver than I would have been otherwise. It made risks feel smaller; it made it possible for me to trust myself a little more. Like any mother and child, we'd had our conflicts, our weaknesses, our outright failures, but there had never been a serious or lasting rift between us. Her faith in me was a safety net I couldn't see until it was gone.

I don't know what I'm going to do without her. Without both of them. *I never deserved them*, I think. *They were wrong to love me.*

But every time I try to hate myself, tell myself that I am a worthless daughter, I swear I can hear her voice in my head. It feels new.

Don't say that, she says. *Don't even think it.*

———

We're nearly two months into the pandemic, but the funeral home representative tells me they've never set up a live stream for a funeral and aren't sure whether they can. *We're looking into it.*

My mother's priest has privacy concerns about filming the service, and adds that it was already very difficult to choose who among my mother's many church friends could attend. Only twenty-five people may be present. An additional person filming, he points out, "will take a place that could have gone to another mourner."

I catch my breath in a painful gasp and let the silence stretch. I don't want to get angry. I don't have the energy for it, or for smoothing things over afterward. Mom's church had been her home, the parish community her family. When she got too sick to work, they took up a collection to help, which my proud mother accepted because she knew it was a gift of love and not charity. I'll always be grateful to her church for being there for her when I wasn't, doing what I couldn't.

But I'm her only child.

"You have four spots you wouldn't have if my husband, my kids, and I were able to be there," I say at last. "Can't you just think of the person filming as taking my place?"

There's a brief pause. "Of course," he says, sounding

somewhat chastened. "You're absolutely right. I'm sure we can work something out."

—

When I'm not talking with the priest, or the funeral home, or the home health-care agency that tells me to please watch for at least two more bills, I wait for the darkness to close over me. The way it did in the months after my father died. The way it did last Christmas, when I realized it was likely my last with my mother. I wait for that terrible voice to whisper that I was useless to my parents, and so my life, too, is useless.

This time it doesn't come.

So many people are dying, every day, during the pandemic. The whole world is grieving. I think of what I gave up, what my mother gave up, so that I could try to keep my family and my kids safe. I have never felt pain like this, but living, I realize, is something I do want.

—

Friends reach out to check on me. I respond to their texts, but I can't seem to pick up the phone when they call. I start to feel nauseated every time it rings; my heart rate spikes, and though I worry that I must appear ungrateful, I cannot bring myself to answer or call back. I finally realize that I have developed a deep and reflexive anxiety about phone calls, because every call for weeks has been about my mother's coming death. My husband starts carrying my phone for me, letting me know when it's something I need to respond to.

Our house begins to fill with food and flowers and gifts. My friends record and send video condolences. My sister sends soup and rolls and cookies and socks. Sympathy cards arrive from all over the country; from Oregon, my parents' friends write and share memories. *Your mom was the first person to greet me when I joined the parish. Your dad could always make my kids laugh. Thank you for sharing them with us.* Candles are lit, Masses are offered, trees are planted in my mother's honor. I am given homemade cookies, handmade jewelry, favorite poems written on elegant card stock. I quickly lose track of who has sent and done what, and wish I had kept a better list. I know everyone is doing this because they want me to feel that, even sequestered at home, I'm not alone. While our losses and disappointments and absences are our own, in the midst of a pandemic killing thousands of people each day, no one needs to dig very deep to understand what my family and I are going through.

And yet there are days when I can barely get a handle on it myself, and it feels as though my mother's death took place in another timeline, another universe. In my darkest moments, I worry that the worst of my grief lies ahead—lurking, waiting for me, biding its time. Loss in this time of distancing and isolation can feel like skirting the borders of a deep, dense forest that is still largely unknown and unexplored; if it hurts this much now, at the outermost edge of the woods, I wonder what will happen if I am ever able to venture in.

———

In my mother's parish, it is the priest who speaks about the deceased midway during the funeral liturgy, and I know this is what she would have wanted—the traditional, the familiar.

Still, sometimes I find myself mentally composing a eulogy of sorts, words I might have offered if I'd been asked. *In my life, my mother's care is like the foundation of a recipe,* I could say. *I have made it my own—I might change some of the steps, some of the components—but no matter what, you will always see her influence in what I do, in the final result.* On and on this goes, one lacking metaphor after another; in the end, I'm dissatisfied with everything I come up with, and think to myself that it's just as well I won't be invited to speak.

I feel crushed beneath the weight of the knowledge that if I'd lost Mom at any other time, it would have been possible for me to be with her at the end; to attend her funeral; to witness and fully participate in all the customs we observe when someone we love dies. These rituals can still leave us feeling incomplete, of course, but they can also act as signposts, guiding us from one phase of mourning to another. When my father died, being at his funeral with my mother, seeing his casket lowered into the ground, telling stories and crying with others who loved him were all things that helped me to acknowledge the loss, talk about it with others, feel and begin to process and live with it. I had thought of these rites as universal hallmarks of grief, belonging to all who must say goodbye to loved ones. I had not realized that mourning in the known or expected way could also be a luxury, a privilege, one that might disappear in a moment.

When I lose my mother, it's without these familiar touchstones. I have to watch her funeral from my living room couch, squished between my husband and children, the same couch where we'd crowded around my phone for our last call with her. We've all dressed up a little, even though no one on the other end of the live feed can see us. I suppose I just cannot imagine attending my mother's funeral, even remotely, in the same sweatpants I've been living in for weeks.

I recognize the prayers, the songs we heard at my father's funeral. I see some of the same faces, too, although they are harder to identify when masked. The cameras are positioned so that we always see her lying in the casket her friend Luke made for her, a twin of the one he made my father. She is nearly as pale as the white garment that drapes her from neck to toe, and there is an Orthodox cross and an icon of Saint Gabriel the Archangel in the casket with her. My twelve-year-old and I cry at the shock of seeing her face, so small and still, not my mother's face at all.

We listen as her priest speaks about what a strong, faithful, and beloved woman she was. He mentions that my mother died the day before what would have been my parents' forty-seventh wedding anniversary—which means, he says, that they spent their anniversary together. *May their memories be eternal.* I look across the room, where my parents' wedding photo sits on the piano, my young father in his powder-blue tuxedo, my younger mother with her white gown, lace cap, and an enormous bouquet of white daisies.

There is a live feed from the cemetery as well, so we are able to see her burial and graveside service. But afterward there is no gathering or mercy meal, no hugs and fellowship with family and friends, no stories exchanged through laughter and tears—all things my mother would have loved. The feed cuts to black, and then it's just us, alone in our house, thousands of miles away.

I look up and see one of our neighbors walking up our

driveway with a vase of garden-grown snapdragons, deep purple and fuchsia and white. I wave to her and bring the flowers inside, and my family and I sit down to eat the lunch Dan has prepared. We don't see or speak to anyone else for the rest of the day.

———

For me, grief is like waking up every day in a different house. I feel as though I ought to know my way around by now——I have been grieving for my father for more than two years——but find that I am continually losing my bearings, struggling to learn the layout anew. I will walk through a door in my mind that I didn't even notice the day before, trip over a memory I've relived a thousand times, and it's as if I were seeing the space around me, breathing in this hushed loneliness, for the first time.

I try to talk to my husband and children about my mother, but soon stop. It is too much of an effort; it feels forced. I have to explain so much before they can understand, and even then there's no way for them to join me in the past. It's the same when I bring up my father or my grandmother. The three people who saw me through my childhood, who remember best what I was like as a baby and a little girl, are gone, and now I carry these stories and memories alone. Three deaths, one composite lump of grief.

"How are you feeling?" my favorite cousin asks me one day. He calls and texts often to check on me, the sort of kindness I'd expect from him. He didn't spend a great deal of time with my parents when he was growing up, but at least he remembers their outlines; he knew them as long as he's known me.

I hear myself saying, "It's like being unadopted."

And yet when someone else says, "Welcome to the shittiest club, the motherless club," it's as if someone has struck me. I imagine my mother's face if she heard anyone call me that. *She would be livid*, I think, and the sound I hear coming from my throat is not quite a laugh, but it is close.

A friend points out that my parents' deaths were inversions of each other, from the duration of their illnesses to my ability to provide practical assistance to whether and how I was able to be with them and engage in public mourning after they died. *Put them both together*, I think, *and I got to experience one whole loss as expected*. Is it any wonder that I often struggle to experience these losses as distinct, to grieve for each of them separately? I have never had enough time.

——

Sometimes I almost imagine that there must exist some ideal state of mourning, a perfectly balanced equation that will allow me to miss my parents, feel sad that they are gone, but remain myself, somehow, in control, anchored in the life I have to continue living without them. But of course no perfect balance exists. There will be days ahead that are all joy and days that are all grief—right now, I know only the latter—and an infinite number of combinations and feelings in between. I will control none of it. I can only let it be what it's going to be.

So I go back to work, far sooner than I'd like. I return to therapy, though my sessions are now remote. My husband is still doing the lion's share of the parenting, but I do my part to help our younger child get through the virtual school day, resuming my place at her side during her language-arts lessons. I try to keep alive all the plants I received as sympathy gifts, buying delicate stakes and clips for the orchids. I take long walks by the creek near our house, picking my way along the bank slowly and carefully, as if there are snags and hidden holes everywhere instead of a smooth trail. I wear the softest clothes I own, along with my mother's rings, the ones she gave to me before she died.

I've been back at work for a few weeks when a co-worker asks me where I'm most looking forward to traveling *once this is all over.*

In the long silence that follows, I hear them apologize. They know that it is too late for the only trip I care about, the visit I wasn't able to make. Our conversation moves on, mercifully, and I am not angry, though I cannot stop think-ing about their question—about how it would feel to be able to look ahead, without fear, without this choking grief, to whomever I will see and whatever I will do and whoever I will be if a safer world ever opens up. I wonder if, no matter what lies ahead, I'll spend the rest of my life looking backward, re-living the endless days and nights when my mother was dying and I couldn't be with her.

22

THE PRIORITY MAIL BOXES BEGIN ARRIVING IN JUNE. Packed and shipped by my aunts, each box is stuffed with photos, documents, correspondence, religious items, knick-knacks, jewelry. Sometimes I let them sit for days before I feel able to sift through the contents. Sometimes I tear them open at once, hoping to find items to show my family.

One holds my mother's jewelry boxes, her high school diploma, her senior photo, and the stub of a ticket to a Simon & Garfunkel concert she'd once told me about, her eyes shining: *It was the best live concert I've ever seen.* In another, amid old family photographs I have never seen before, I find Mom's wallet and driver's license, a bill from the attorney who'd represented my parents in my adoption, and a copy of the will she had written only months before. There's a wooden box full of bead necklaces: black and white, turquoise, yellow, royal blue, celadon green. *Did she wear all of these?* I wonder. *Any of them?* The only necklace I can recall seeing around her neck, at least in recent years, is her sterling-silver Orthodox cross with the dark blue inlay.

My older daughter picks out a necklace of aubergine beads and gives it to her little sister. Rummaging through another box, I don't see what happens or how the string snaps; I only hear a sudden shower of beads hitting the floor. The girls pick them up together, sneaking slightly worried looks at me, but I'm not upset. There must be a dozen strings of beads in the box; one won't be missed. Though I know we'll never wear them, I can't bring myself to get rid of them, or anything else that belonged to her or my dad. The boxes, once opened, pile up in my office.

I find notes I wrote to my mom when I was five, large print crammed into hand-drawn hearts: *Dear Mom, Well, how are you? How was work? Fine I hope! Sarra and me had a good time. Well, bye, love you.* I find cards made for her de-cades later, by my own kids: *Dear Grandma, Thank you for the gifts and treats! We miss you. We hope we can visit you soon.* I find old report cards, paintings, postcards we sent to her, a heart-shaped cardboard picture frame I decorated in either second or fourth grade by gluing hundreds of painted pasta shells into place, just so. I find my father's Cleveland Browns shot glass, which I recall him using as a toothpick holder. I find a letter from my mother to my father, trying to mend a rift after a fight, and it feels like something I should never have seen.

Toward the bottom of one box, I find Mom's brand-new passport, the one she had renewed for her planned trip to Greece. She was going to go with her friends the year Dad died, and then the year after, but both times cancer ruined her plans. Her new passport sat in the envelope it had come in, in a box on top of her filing cabinet, until it was retrieved, packed up in a box, and sent to me. I wonder if her friends will go without her, perhaps make the trip in her memory.

Even after she began hospice care, she would say things like *I think I'm feeling better than last week. Maybe next week I'll try to walk again.* If sheer stubbornness could have kept her alive, she would have lived to be a hundred. She deserved more time to mourn, and to fight, and to figure out who she was and what she wanted her life to be after Dad was gone. It would have been a long and painful process, the work of years, but I know that she would have done it. She would have found her way. She would have gone to Greece.

—

Forty days after her death, Mom's priest and her friends visit her grave and pray a Panikhida, an abbreviated memorial service, for her soul. That same day, I receive her prayer book, sent to me by Elizabeth the week before.

The book was my mother's daily companion for years, and it shows; the cover is lovingly worn, threadbare at the corners and along the spine, its gold and white placeholder ribbons beginning to fray at the tips. My mother prayed several times a day: in the morning and evening, at every meal, before she went to sleep. I can hardly remember the last time I prayed the way she did—wholeheartedly, trustingly, sure that God was listening and would never fail to act for her good and the good of those she loved, even if he did so in ways she could not understand.

When I open the book to a random page, the first prayer I see is the Prayer for a Deceased Parent. I think of how often this page must have been read, how many times my mother must have faithfully said this prayer for my grandfather. Did she have a chance to say it for my grandmother? I don't share her unyielding faith, but I have always found it easier to pray for others than for myself, and I know that Mom would want me to pray for her—how well I remember her telling me, *You'd better remember to pray for me when I'm dead!* Somehow this charge feels more important than my doubt.

Remember, O Lord, the souls of Thy servants who have departed in sleep, my parents, and all my relatives according to the flesh; forgive them every transgression, voluntary and involuntary; grant them the Kingdom and a part in Thy eternal joys, and the delight of Thy blessed and everlasting life. Grant, O Lord, remission of all sins to our Fathers, Brothers and Sisters departed in the faith and hope of resurrection, and grant them memory eternal.

The phrase *according to the flesh* trips me up a bit. Neither my adoptive parents nor any of my other known deceased family were my blood relations; I'd been raised to believe that our love and our souls were what counted. I skip that line and read the rest of the words with intention. I can't say whether God hears me. Deep in an unguarded corner of my heart, I feel that my mother does.

———

I don't have to learn how to be fully in the world without her. There is no way to jump back into my old life, no pressure to go out every day and pretend that things are normal for anyone else's benefit. We're still in a pandemic, in a kind of forced suspension. I stay home with my family, and we continue to mourn in our own time, our own space, our own ways.

Much as I want the pandemic to end, I find that I'm almost thankful to avoid any semblance of a normal life. I suspect I'm not the only person in mourning who finds even the possibility of "normal" to be an utterly foreign concept; who wonders how it will feel to face not just one place, but every place, without the person I've lost. Perhaps this is the opposite of that searching phase of grief I've heard about, when you imagine that you can somehow find and recover your loved one who died—I know that no matter where I go now, she won't be found.

Here at home, the territory of loss does not change: I begin to understand how my grief fills this space; I know its height and its breadth. Every room holds memories of it. *This is where I had my last conversation with my mother. This is where I got the call telling me that she was gone. This is where I livestreamed her funeral.* This is where I lost her, but it is also the last place I had her, had a living parent at all. Try as I might, I'm unable to shake the feeling that as long as I am here, I am still with her, keeping my vigil in the only way I can.

Grief is a chasm, one I can lose myself in without trying. And yet it's not quite the unyielding abyss I feared it would be. I thought they would feel farther away—that they would both be lost to me, and that it was what I deserved.

But now, sometimes, I feel they are so close, as if they were only in the next room, as if one of them might hear me if I called. It's not a presence, exactly. But not an absence, either.

I don't know where my mother is, *if* she is. I don't know the shape or form, weight or depth of her existence now. I know that some part of her isn't gone, because I feel her love and experience her care like a living thing. I hear her voice speaking to me. And though my father felt so far from me after he died, he no longer feels so distant, lost beyond my reach—it's as if she has given a part of him back to me now that they are wherever they are, together, my ancestors by love and choice if not by blood.

———

In October, on what would have been my mother's sixty-ninth birthday, I write her a letter and buy a nice meal to eat at home with my family—nothing fancy, nothing my mom had ever made for me, just something I know she would have enjoyed. (She always, until her final days, ate quickly and with much gusto, a trait I'm sure I got from her.) I can't visit her grave, with the headstone I chose to match my dad's, but I send flowers to the cemetery. I order them from the same florist who designed my mother's memorial flowers, and she promises to use the same colors. The two arrangements are made in different seasons, with different flowers in bloom, so of course they cannot be exactly the same. Nor can a livestreamed funeral provide the same experience, the same companionship or comfort, as one you're able to attend in person. But neither this life-changing loss nor the depth of gratitude I feel because I had her as a parent can be undermined by the unforeseen, by disease, or by distance. She was my mother. I will miss her forever. In this way, both her absence and my grief are precisely what they would have been, even in an ordinary time.

23

MY PARENTS MOVED INTO THEIR MANUFACTURED HOME the same year my husband and I moved to North Carolina for his graduate program. I found out they were moving when my mother called and asked me what I wanted to do with my *stuff*, meaning everything that hadn't fit in two suitcases and four media-mail boxes when I went to college. Most of my childhood belongings were still stored in my parents' garage. I told her she was welcome to donate, sell, or toss anything she liked, though I harbored a hope of one day retrieving my old dollhouse for my then-theoretical children to play with.

When a friend asked if I minded that my parents were selling the home I'd grown up in, I scoffed. The last person to live in my childhood bedroom hadn't even been me, but a friend of mine—my parents, with typical openhandedness, had let her stay with them rent-free for a year and a half after her own parents kicked her out. There were things about the house I'd been fond of: the sprawling, shady backyard that had once contained my rickety old swing set; my room with its blue walls and bursting bookshelves and my cat's favorite scratching post; the minuscule spare bedroom that I was eventually permitted to turn into a writing space, nearly every square inch filled with our lumpy blue futon and the giant desk I had begged my mother to buy at a yard sale. But I was an adult now, and I couldn't imagine being so attached to that childhood setting that I would fault my parents for moving. It was *their* home, not mine, and they had a right to sell it.

They sounded upbeat about the change: they'd be closer to their church; they'd be in a quieter neighborhood; they'd have a much lower cost of living. Their house had tripled in value since they bought it in 1980, so they stood to make a nice profit. I was pleased for them, but did not entirely understand their decision. They had talked about relocating for as long as I could remember—first to a bigger city like Portland or Seattle, before they reversed course and said they'd like to live farther out in the country. Now they were finally moving, but not to own a patch of land, or to live in an area with more jobs; instead, they'd paid cash for a manufactured home in good condition in a fifty-five-and-over park fifteen minutes up the road. Why, I wondered, weren't they purchasing a larger home with the windfall from the sale?

Though their new house didn't have the two-car garage or the back forty, it had higher ceilings and two full bathrooms instead of one, and the common spaces felt more comfortable and open. The first time Dan and I visited my parents after their move, my mother was almost giddy as she gave us a tour and pointed out the guest room we would be sleeping in. I knew how happy she was to see us, but there was something else in her smile, in the warmth in her voice, that took me a moment to recognize: it was pride. I'd never known her to feel that way about our old place, but she clearly liked this one; slightly cluttered and freshly cleaned for our visit, the house was arranged in a way that pleased her, and my parents owned it free and clear.

———

After my father died, I remember thinking it strange that I had so few objects to remember him by. Mom wound up donating their wedding bands to a church fundraiser, a decision I couldn't understand, but they were hers to donate. "I know it's what Dad would have wanted," she said. "I heard him telling me to let them go."

It's true that my father didn't hold on to many objects for sentimental reasons—with the exception of his old Boy Scout memorabilia, a link to his father and his brother, and the preemie-sized strawberry-print dress my parents had bought for me to wear when they brought me home from the NICU. When I was younger, its size had meant nothing to me, but now that I've had two babies who would never have fit in such a tiny garment, I understand why my father used to take the dress out sometimes and stare at it, shaking his head in wonder. It's terrifying enough becoming a parent, bringing your child home for the first time—I remember feeling shocked as well as nervous, almost tempted to ask the nurse, *Are you really going to let us walk out of here with this baby?*—but in my parents' case, after nearly a decade of infertility, they had walked out of the hospital with a fragile preemie who'd weighed two pounds at birth and still had no eyebrows.

Though I had asked to hear the story of my adoption and homecoming many times, I'd never asked them if they felt anxious on the long drive home, or during that first night with me. Were they naturals, both being one of five kids and early in the birth order, or did they consult family members and books? How long had it taken them to learn what to do? My mother once told me that for months they would get up in the night and check to make sure that I was breathing, my underdeveloped lungs doing their job.

After Dad's funeral, Mom said I should take the strawberry dress. She let me look through his things and claim anything else I wanted. I found one of his Cleveland Browns caps, the tie pin I'd given him one Christmas, and a heavy knit shawl-collar cardigan I remembered him wearing often as he got older and became more sensitive to the cold. The only other item I pocketed was a small black notebook he used to carry around, in which he'd jotted down appointment times, grocery lists, odd notes and reminders for himself. I kept it not for any of the information it contained but because it was comforting to flip through it and see his familiar handwriting.

———

I found the letter from the courthouse in one of the boxes sent to me after my mother died. It was addressed to both my parents, and I had to read it twice before I could understand what it was: a notice confirming their bankruptcy filing. It was from the year after I graduated from college, the year before they sold their old house and moved to the mobile-home park. My father had not been gravely ill yet, and both he and my mother were working at the time. I could only guess that this was the result of insurmountable medical debt from my high school years.

I knew they hadn't lost the house, their cars, all their other assets. Was this one reason why they'd sold their home and opted for a more affordable housing situation? Had they promised to use some of the money from the sale to satisfy their creditors? Whatever the truth was, I would not hear it from them now. I knew why they hadn't told me; I could hear their voices as if they stood before me, hands spread, faces closed. *What could you have done? We didn't want you to worry.*

So often, I had wished that I could do more to help them; my greatest failures, I believed, were as their daughter. I felt as responsible for them as they were for me. But had I been wrong to feel that way? They certainly never saw their burdens as mine to share, instead choosing to shield me from them for as long as they could. They were my parents: they looked after me, not the other way around.

———

The lack of air-conditioning in my childhood home was bearable because we could open our windows at night—except during wildfire season, when we might occasionally suffer and sweat in the hot, tightly sealed rooms of our house. The fires rarely threatened more densely populated areas, and I never worried about them reaching our house. From time to time, we would hear that a friend who lived much farther out from town had to evacuate, but I didn't know anyone who had lost their home to fire. I can remember only a few late summer or early fall days when smoky air settled in the hills and hollows around us, making it impossible to go outside and play.

The land, the climate, and the housing patterns have all changed in the years since I left home. Four months after my mother died, a fire started fifteen minutes from her neighborhood. High winds carried the sparks far afield, allowing the blaze to grow and fan out for miles. Unlike the wildfires I remember from childhood, this one roared parallel to some of the busiest roads in the area, ravaging parkland, businesses, and thousands of homes.

I was shocked to see news of the runaway destruction, although California wildfires had been in the news for weeks, and I'd heard about the terrible air quality in the Bay Area, Seattle, Portland, Vancouver. My home region lacks a major urban center and rarely draws outside media attention. But the damage was too vast to be ignored, and terrifying headlines and images from my parents' tiny town of a few thousand residents soon filled my social media feeds. I checked on friends and acquaintances and tried to call my aunt, who had inherited my parents' house after my mother died. When I didn't get an answer, I texted Paula, who confirmed that she, her husband, and my aunt were safe—and so was Buster. They were all hunkered down at Paula's, in sight of the flames but hoping they wouldn't need to evacuate. They couldn't say whether my parents' home had survived.

Dan and I scoured the internet for local news reports, searching for the name of my parents' park and other nearby landmarks. We watched shaky video footage shot by local residents; paused and zoomed in on aerial video shared by local news outlets, trying to identify my parents' neighborhood. When I stumbled over an article about entire groves of ponderosa pines lost to wildfire, I felt another kind of grief. What if the cemetery had been leveled, too? I pictured the peaceful graveyard, with its hundred-year-old oaks and pines, bare and smoking; my parents' gravestones scorched and illegible. I thought again of their house, their windows facing the mountains, their closets stuffed with clothing and linens and boxes of family photos, their shelves full of books and religious art and my grandmother's glassware and collectibles—was any of it left?

When they sold the house I'd grown up in, the thought of strangers owning it—whether they made it their own, updated and flipped it, or tore it down to build something new—hadn't caused me a moment's distress. I'd never lived in their second Oregon home or grown deeply attached to it, but it was a place that was theirs, a place that held memories of our final visits. Even if all their belongings were gone, the loss was a small one compared with what many in the region were experiencing: people had lost their loved ones, their homes, their livelihoods. Still, I knew that I would grieve if all that remained of my parents' life together was now ash and smoke.

—

Before wildfire season began, I had a video call with a friend who had recently moved to San Francisco. She took the call outside on her balcony, angling her screen to show me the just-barely view of the bay. She looked so cool and comfortable, I tried not to feel envious, sweating in my office even with the air conditioner blasting. "You can always move back out here, you know," she told me with a grin; she knew that I missed the Northwest, its climate and its vast natural beauty, and sometimes dreamed of relocating to one of its cities. One month later, as friends and family throughout the West hunted for giant air filters and worked to seal their homes against smoke, I worried for them and wondered if I could, indeed, go home again.

It would be a week before we learned that my parents' home was still standing. Many of the surrounding neighborhoods were gone. So was the doughnut shop up the road, where I went to buy doughnuts the day after Christmas, and the engraver's shop across the street that had made my parents' matching headstones, and the park where my children used to play and collect pebbles in the creek bed. Much of what burned were manufactured homes and apartment complexes, where seniors and immigrant families and many others on fixed incomes had lived and called home; thousands of people, including many children, were left to scramble for new housing. The land and its residents have yet to fully recover, and of course wildfire season will continue to return each year, threatening what remains and what has been rebuilt.

It feels obscene to call it luck when something precious to you survives amid such widespread devastation. Still, I can't help but feel grateful that the house where my parents lived and died survived. Of all the places they lived together, I think it was their favorite. It was a home they owned outright after so many uncertain years; a home that gave them community. A home they could feel proud of.

24

SINCE I WAS A CHILD, I'VE BEEN ABLE TO WAKE MYSELF UP from dreams. But I find it's hard to leave dreams about my parents, even the nightmares. It's the only time I get to see their faces, hear their voices as I remember them.

In one dream, the night after what would have been my mother's sixty-ninth birthday, I see her standing in the backyard at my grandmother's house—not the last one Grandma lived in, or even the one before that, but the one she and my grandfather bought when they moved from California to southern Oregon to be closer to my parents. It was a small ranch house like ours, plain white with brown shutters, but filled with the magic of my grandmother's imagination—she was an avid gardener, dancer, and fisherwoman who collected crystals and kites and music boxes—and the smell of her delicious cooking. I loved playing in her backyard, where she had a gazebo and a rose trellis, a decorative windmill and a birdbath, a giant vegetable garden and another for flowers, a cherry tree and a wild blackberry bush. In the dream, my mother is young, younger than I can remember her being, happy and healthy, setting up lawn chairs for us on the grass.

Sometimes, when I dream about my parents, it's comforting; I can touch them and hug them. Sometimes the dreams are painful; they're angry with me and refuse to tell me why, or they're sick and I cannot help. One night, I dream that I'm unable to reach my dying mother because I am being held in prison for a crime I didn't commit. I beg my jailers, anyone, to please let me go and see her, but am only allowed a single call.

A few nights ago, I dreamed that we were in a cabin in the mountains, about to sit down to dinner. There might have been other people in the dream, but I only remember talking to my mom, sitting across from her at a farmhouse table, unburdening myself the way I used to do when I was younger and she was the only person I wanted to talk to. I was worried about my younger daughter, I told her. Due to her disability and her specific learning needs, she requires significant support and accommodations in order to make progress at school. We've had to fight hard for what she is legally entitled to, and it has been harder than ever since the start of the pandemic. Her educators this year seem to have given up on her, and I am no longer certain how best to advocate for her.

Though my mom did not always understand my younger child's disability, she saw and loved and seemed to understand something fundamentally important about her. It never would have occurred to her to wish that either of my children was different; they were her grandchildren, which meant they were the most wonderful children in the world, just as they were. She allowed herself to not fret, to simply *be* with them: fully present, fully accepting. Her happiest hours were spent watching them read or play; no matter what they did, she found them both perfect and endlessly entertaining. She never needed an agenda when she visited us, never needed them to do anything or be anything other than themselves.

When I was at my most anxious, fretting about one or both of my kids, Mom would always tell me to relax, take a deep breath, stop worrying. *The girls are going to be okay.* It was no empty, unthinking reassurance she offered; she believed it, every time. I couldn't understand her certainty, and sometimes, I admit, resented it—she was a parent, too, and as anxious as I was. Didn't she understand that it was impossible for me to let go of my fears, lay down my burdens?

Now I would give almost anything to hear her tell me not to worry again. In my dream the other night, as I talked with her about my daughter, I could feel her hand pressing down on mine, the warmth of her fingers, the grain of the wooden table at which we sat. I could hear her voice, as clear as it was in life. *You can tell me all about it*, she said. *And then you'll figure out how to help her, like you always do.* When I woke, it occurred to me that perhaps my mind is trying to mother me, now that my mother is gone.

25

AT AROUND EIGHT BY TEN, MY OFFICE IS THE SMALLEST
of our small bedrooms, squished between the master bedroom and my older daughter's room. I claimed it as my work
space when we moved into this, the first residence of my
adult life that has felt semipermanent. I pushed an old table
up against the room's only window, pleased to find that during the day, at least, there is no need for a lamp. We painted
the walls a soft blue green that reminds me of sea glass, and I
hung up original art and carefully arranged the bookshelves. I
hadn't had a dedicated writing space all to myself, with a door
I could close, since I took over the spare bedroom in my childhood home. For our first two years in the house, the study was
my primary work space, the backdrop for all my video meetings, the place where I went to brainstorm and to write.

Then we got a dog, and I pretty much stopped working
there altogether.

For years, whenever one of our children asked us if we
could get a puppy, Dan or I would offer up a vague response:

Maybe someday, when you're old enough to help. Several friends who also had autistic children had gotten them therapy dogs—mostly Labradors or goldendoodles—and we had thought about doing the same. Both of us had grown up with dogs and cats and were generally pro-pets, but we also knew how much extra work it would mean.

Then came the pandemic. Sometime between my mother's funeral in the spring and back-to-school that never quite happened in the fall, *maybe* gave way to *yes* and *someday* became *as soon as possible*. Saying yes to the dog was very much about saying yes to our kids in the worst year of their lives. They'd lost so much in such a brief space of time: another grandparent, visits with family, familiar routines, a sense of stability and safety. Their schools were still closed, which meant they spent five hours a day in front of their Chromebook screens, being reminded to sit up straight and keep their cameras on. Their world had shrunk to the four walls of our house, our yard, and the neighborhood we meandered through day after day. We knew that we were luckier than many. We were trying our best. But none of us were doing well, and the first long pandemic winter was on the way. This dog, I decided, was going to be the family comfort animal.

The kids picked out a name together and refused to consider any others. It was my lap that Peggy curled up on to sleep during the drive home, firmly rejecting the blanket-and-newspaper-lined cardboard box we'd brought with us. By the time she came along to throw our entire household into joyful chaos, several more families we knew had gotten dogs. One went "just to look" at a litter of puppies and wound up bringing one home on the same day we got Peggy, without so much as a dog bed or food bowl ready. Holdouts teased us for giving their children fuel for their own pandemic pet campaigns. "Way to make it that much harder for the rest of us," one friend said. "I want my kid to meet your puppy, but also my kid should *never* meet your puppy."

We had no regrets, even on days when Peggy woke us before dawn and soiled the floor every twenty minutes. She followed us from room to room, searching for someone to cuddle with when she wanted to sleep—I'd never met a needier being, yet she seemed convinced that she was taking care of us, not the other way around. She would often nap under the kids' desks during their endless school Zoom days, near enough to be stealthily petted.

One day I came into the living room to find our twelve-pound puppy exuberantly chasing my older child in circles around our coffee table, and I realized it was the first I'd heard her deep belly laugh in weeks. Nearly every other time I'd witnessed someone's happiness or glee in the months since my mother's death, I felt as though I were viewing it through a thick sheet of glass—though I might smile or laugh along, the emotion itself remained indistinct, inaccessible to me, something I could see and remember but not feel, at least not fully. The joy on my daughter's face as Peggy scampered after her stood out so clear and sharp and bright, it was as if I could reach out and grab ahold of it.

———

I don't remember when or why I first began to pay attention to my mother's anxiety. At some point I realized that talking with her sometimes made *me* more anxious, but it wasn't clear to me why; like me, she was someone I thought of as a worrier, but it wasn't as if she were always catastrophizing when we talked. She had a hard time with silence, I noticed, and couldn't help but try to fill it, which sometimes meant a jarring topic shift or slightly nervous joke. It was difficult for her to sit still. She picked at her nails. When these things annoyed me, it was because I knew that I had the exact same tendencies.

A few months before my mom died, my therapist pointed out that the level of anxiety I experience isn't typical, either. I felt no need to deny this; as in my mother's case, it seemed obvious to me why I was anxious. One of my parents had died, and the other now had terminal cancer. I was caring for my family and working all the time and trying to promote a book. I wasn't taking care of myself. Was it any wonder that my neck felt as if it were made of granite, that I was grinding my teeth so much I needed to replace my night guard, that I frequently found myself unable to fall asleep?

She allowed that I certainly had cause to worry. But what else did I worry about, besides my family? And before my parents had gotten sick, what symptoms of anxiety had I noticed?

As a child, when the bullying was at its worst, I went through a period of twisting and twirling my hair, sometimes pulling it out. As a teenager, I had experienced months of insomnia, which still came back to plague me now and then. A decade ago, I'd had a three-month headache and gone to see a neurologist. "Women carry so much stress in their bodies," he told me. "Of course, it could also be hormones." He prescribed a low dose of antianxiety medication, which I took for a few months, tapered as instructed, and then forgot about.

On any given day, I can easily think of a dozen worst-case scenarios to warn my friends and loved ones about. My husband is rear-ended on the highway, and for weeks I'm afraid when he has to drive anywhere. My daughters go swimming, and I can't resist a last-minute lecture about pool safety that they've heard many times before. *No running!* I always want to believe that anticipating the disaster, trying to predict it, will somehow allow me to control it or even prevent it from occurring. I am *watchful*, I've often thought. I am *prepared*.

In my mother's final months, I had little time to think about or dwell on my own physical or mental state. When I finally noticed the hard, aching knot in my chest, I assumed it was because I was angry and heartbroken over what was happening to her. But the chest tightness was a symptom of anxiety—like the tension headaches that came and went, the perpetual stiffness in my neck and shoulders, the faint twitch under my left eye, the unsettled stomach that sometimes made it hard to eat. I wasn't having the sort of breakdown I'd once imagined, one announced in more obvious signs of distress: trembling, shortness of breath, a sudden elevated heart rate, dizziness or weakness or chills. Not until the pandemic hit and I suddenly felt like a rat trapped in a maze, frantically circling and unable to escape, did it occur to me that I might be experiencing a constant, low-level panic attack, a slow but inexorable spiral from which there would be no escape so long as my mother suffered and I could not get to her. And even then, I kept working, taking care of my children, doing what needed to be done.

I cannot recall every symptom I've ever experienced, every moment when I have felt the heave and pull of anxiety in my head or my chest or my stomach, but I suspect that I have probably always lived with it, this inheritance from both my families. I don't feel it in my body so often now; the physical symptoms crested while my mom was dying, and began to recede after. Sometimes I think that my anxiety is more easily triggered in the wake of my parents' deaths. Or maybe it is only that I can now recognize it for what it is, no longer overlooking or dismissing it when it returns. It is like a dog attempting to warn me, barking at something I cannot quite see in the dark—I might be tempted to ignore it in the hope that it stops, but have learned that if I acknowledge it instead, give it some of my attention, it may quiet, its warning delivered.

It has taken time to understand the ways in which grief can interact with and feed my anxiety; sometimes, I think, I lean too far into it, let my mind run away with worrying and planning, so that grief is not all that I feel. When my thoughts are churning, trying to find some way to avert catastrophe and wish us into a different, better world, I don't have to focus on the fact that I live in this one, where my heart is still broken.

———

I wasn't thinking about my anxiety when we decided to get a dog; I was thinking about my family and the fact that we had never been more in need of comfort and a limitless source of uncomplicated love. More than once, I thought of what my mother said when she got Buster: *He's good for me. He gets me out of the house. No matter how I feel or what I want, I have to take him for his walk. I'm never alone anymore.* In the last weeks of her life, Buster was always with her, curled up beside her in the hospital bed. My aunt takes care of him now, in the house he used to share with my mom, and I like to think that he remembers her as well as he can—the rooms may yet hold traces of her that a dog's sharp nose can sniff out. I'm thankful that he was with her until the end.

Now full grown at one year old, Peggy remains a puppy—curious, affectionate, high-energy, ready to greet and be devoted to anyone who crosses her path. Her name is forever bouncing off the walls of our house: an excited greeting when we come home to find her waiting, tail wagging; a grumble of irritation when she does something naughty; a murmur of appreciation when she curls up next to us to offer comfort. She isn't allowed in my office, because I don't know that I could trust her exuberant bulk or wide-swinging tail around the breakables there, and suspect she might also try to nose some of my books down from the shelves. Now I write at the kitchen table, with Peggy napping at my feet.

Though I'm highly allergic to most dogs, no one has spent more time cuddling with her, ruffling her silky-soft fur and scratching her ears, than I have. I end most days on the couch or the floor, her head in my lap, and these moments never fail to slow my anxious thoughts and soothe my heart. I think she immediately recognized that I was broken and needed her, which could be why the two of us have such a deep soul bond. (Or it could be because she has learned that I have the freest hand with the dog biscuits, who can say.) I don't want to say that she saved us from our grief, because neither loss nor healing works that way. But with her, we've been able to access a kind of effortless happiness we hadn't known for a long time. She has given our weary, grieving family another place to put our love, a shared focus that isn't all about what we've lost, and I am often reminded that this, too, is part of mourning: trying to find new joy where we can.

Pets represent an ongoing expense, and there were many years when it would have been easier if my parents hadn't had to pay for their care and feeding. I think Dad would have gladly skipped the experience: when we had a dog in the house, it was because my mother loved them. I grew up hearing stories about the family pets who'd chased her around the farm growing up. Casey, a basset hound/beagle we got when I was two, was named for her uncle Casimir; when he died a few days before I left for college, it felt like the end of my childhood, and no one cried more than my mom. In several of my favorite photos of her, she has her arms wrapped around one of her cherished pups, and though I can't always name the year or the pup, I can see my mother happy, and remember how her cares and worries, even her fear of dying, had been eased when she had a faithful dog at her side.

We often talk about how much my mom would have loved Peggy. She would have sent her toys and treats, offered her another warm lap on her visits, peppered us with questions about her training and her habits bad and good. She would have loved watching her romp with the kids, and probably laughed to see how much I depend on her. "Maybe Grandma knows about her," my older daughter suggested one day. "I'm sure she still knows about the really important things."

26

WHEN MY FATHER TURNED FORTY, HIS CO-WORKERS AT the pizza parlor, who'd hung black balloons and crepe-paper streamers from the light fixtures, presented him with a cake covered in deep, dark fudge frosting, OVER THE HILL written in thin white icing. Dad was always delighted by a joke, the darker, the better, and I remember him laughing as he cut slices for everyone. On my fortieth birthday, no one made jokes about my age or my mortality. Even I spared little thought for the number itself. The only milestone that seemed to matter was that it was my first birthday without both my parents.

Sometimes, though, I feel more vulnerable in my own skin because my parents are gone, as if I am a person to whom anything might happen now that they are no longer here to guard me—"To take / the first blows / on their shoulders," as poet Linda Pastan wrote. It doesn't help to know I've entered the decade when they both faced different life-changing diagnoses. Routine physicals, unheard of for much of my youth, have become a new source of anxiety. My doctor orders blood work and screenings, noting "baselines," values that could be higher or lower, things we should keep our eye on. I experience pain that drives me to seek out physical therapy, massage therapy, my heating pad, my value-sized bottle of ibuprofen. Friends near me in age listen to me complain and then share their own symptoms, aches, therapies, diagnoses. I imagine telling my mother that I find aging empowering in one sense, humbling in another—*I don't mind the number, it's everything else*—and I can almost hear her laughing at me: *Don't be ridiculous, you're still young.* How much of a difference would it make now, I wonder, if she were here to talk to about this? Would aging feel any easier if I could also watch her grow old?

I remember telling her that my doctor and I were watching my blood sugar. By the time I crossed a line I'd been dancing along for years since having children—I barely squeaked through the three-hour-fasting glucose test during both pregnancies, and my sugar never returned to normal after that—she had so little time left, and whether she would be upset or remind me of what Dad had gone through or offer nothing but support, I couldn't bear to tell her that I'd been diagnosed with the disease responsible for his death. There was no opportunity to slow down and process what it would mean for me; the truth was, I didn't know. I took my medication, tried to follow my doctor's advice, tried not to think about it otherwise. This was easier than it sounds, because I did not feel sick, and because all my worry was for my mother.

My father was sixty-seven when he died. My mother was

sixty-eight. I tell myself it is irrational to think that their fates might in any way reflect or predestine mine—every bit of my genetic code is built from others. And yet sometimes it is impossible for me to imagine living longer than they did, making it to seventy and beyond. How could I live to see an age my parents never saw? I can see myself traveling as far as they did, but no further.

A few months after I turned forty, I left the publisher I'd been with for five years. I loved my editorial work and my team, but grief and overwork had worn me down in ways I was no longer able to ignore. I had spent the last decade working my way up, feeling that I always had to do *more*, say yes to everything, to publish my own writing and attain professional roles that rarely seemed to go to people like me. I had worked through a book release and two tours, a pandemic, the deaths of both my parents, emergency after emergency; I'd started skipping meals, editing at all hours of the day and night, writing through the weekend, an-swering emails while on vacation and bereavement leave. There was always more and more to do, and everyone else at my level worked all the time, too, so how could I do otherwise?

Now I write full time. I know how unexpectedly the trajectory of a creative career may shift, and I take nothing for granted, but for the moment I can support myself this way, and I am glad to no longer cram all my writing into the narrow margins of my life. I still drive myself hard to meet deadlines, set my own needs aside for the sake of my work. There are afternoons when my husband will bring me a sandwich and a water bottle in the middle of a marathon writing session, and I will realize that I haven't had a bite of food or a sip of water all day; there are evenings and weekends when everyone else in my family is relaxing, enjoying precious time together, while I sit at my computer. But I am slowly learning how to work with this body I have, trying to listen to what it needs rather than demanding it do what I want. I am learning how to say no if there is no way to yes without sacrificing something vital. I am trying to learn how to rest when I must, because writing is work I love and want to do, and the choices I make, day to day, year to year, are what will allow me to sustain it over a lifetime.

I have found similar lessons in learning to take better care of myself and learning to live with grief—both have forced me to gradually awaken to specific needs and limitations, to accept them as reality, and remember that I am not the machine I used to pretend I was. I also know that none of these lessons would matter were I unsupported, unable to make healthy choices or access the treatment and care I need. I often think of the medical care my father couldn't get, the help he was denied. He was likely diabetic for some time before he was diagnosed; he only went to the doctor once he was experiencing symptoms. He told me that he didn't feel sick at all—until suddenly he did.

Now I understand how hard it can be to believe that you have a serious illness when you cannot easily see evidence of it. Like anxiety, diabetes runs in both my families—an adoptive parent and an adoptive grandparent, a biological parent and a biological grandparent, and these are only the generations I know about. My doctor is always telling me how fortunate I am that we caught it early. I know that much of how I'll fare in the coming decades will come down to genes, and luck, and the choices I make. My grief for my father is also a constant reminder of what I could lose.

———

My mother died two weeks after my thirty-ninth birthday, the week after Mother's Day, and so May, once my favorite month, is now the toughest for me to get through. I struggle through April, too: watching winter retreat and the trees bud and blossom; celebrating Easter, my mother's favorite holiday, though to her it was Pascha; all the time, dreading May, when everything will sound and look and smell exactly as it did when she died.

Mom must have been the one who first told me that emerald is my birthstone—maybe when she bought me one of those cheap little adjustable birthstone rings from the standing cardboard display near the register at the drugstore after I begged, or when she gave me a rosary strung with shiny green beads, made of plastic but cut to sparkle like crystal, the day I made my first Communion. Her birthstone was opal, and she had two opal rings, an opal pendant, and an opal bracelet, all of which came to me after she died. I have bought myself several more pieces of opal jewelry since then, all beautiful, one-of-a-kind rings that remind me of her. After opals, Mom loved emeralds best, because she associated them with me.

The day before my fortieth birthday—my first without her—a package arrived from Oregon. Inside was a card from my aunt and a small cloth gift bag, and inside the bag was a plain white jewelry box containing a beautiful ring, chosen for me by my mother: a deep green emerald set in gleaming white gold, flanked by two small round diamonds. *Your mom always loved you in emeralds—her May baby*, my aunt had written. *She would often talk about you turning forty, expressing disbelief at how fast the time had gone.*

My mother was always thrilled and more than a bit smug when she found the perfect present for someone, whether it was a big-ticket item or a gag gift. Birthdays and Christmases growing up were special not because we had a ton of presents but because she had chosen and wrapped each one. She would beam as she watched everyone open their gifts, because she knew that amid the bargain-basement or secondhand-shop finds would be hidden gems we would love and treasure. I remember how pleased she was watching me open the music box that looked like an open storybook and played the song "Camelot," the pale blue glass perfume bottle she'd found at an antiques shop, the delicate gold cross necklace I would wear for years.

When I saw the emerald, I knew she wouldn't have splurged on such a ring for herself. But by the time she picked it out for me, she knew that she was dying. She didn't feel a need to save money for herself, for retirement, for the trip she'd once hoped to take to Greece.

When I wear the ring now, I imagine her smiling; telling me how good it looks on my hand; sharing how she went to shop after shop, looking for the perfect ring, and when she saw this one—*I just knew.* I never expected Mom to find a way to send me a birthday gift from beyond the grave. But perhaps I shouldn't be so shocked, because if I know anything about my mother, it's that she gave the best of everything she had to others—to me, especially—and that she was always, always thinking of me. I can't help but believe that she may yet find other ways to surprise me.

27

THINGS MY MOTHER LEFT ME

Three wooden jewelry boxes, mostly filled with earrings she had stopped wearing after her ear piercings closed

Pictures of every house she lived in

A raku vase and bowl made by a friend

A pink needlepoint heart I made for her in grade school

Every card, note, and drawing my daughters ever sent to her

Her high school yearbook

Her black-and-white senior portrait, wallet-sized

Her replacement wedding band, bought after she donated my parents' original wedding bands to the church

Half a dozen small colored glass vases collected by my grandmother

My father's favorite Cleveland Browns sweatshirt and his bucket hat

Her impeccable taste in musicals and mystery novels

Her stubbornness

Her anxiety

A habit of silently reciting Hail Marys when I'm worried and can't fall asleep

A belief that my children will be okay

An expansive definition of the word *okay*

A model of forgiveness

The hope that I can be half the parent she was

Her icon of the Angel at the Tomb (*Why do you seek the living among the dead?*)

Her love of the ocean

28

AS THE FIRST ANNIVERSARY OF MY MOTHER'S DEATH draws near, I become obsessed with finding a beach to spend it on. *Finding* a beach, because our go-to spot doesn't allow dogs. Dan and I scroll through listings of rental houses on unfamiliar shores, oceanfront properties only—because when it's rainy or cold or you're done with the beach for the day or engrossed in that novel you're finally going to read, you still want to be able to sit in some warm, dry place and sip your coffee and watch and listen to the sea, expansive, ever changing, soothing as nothing else is.

The first time he and I went to a North Carolina beach together, he marveled at the change in me. I talked and moved more slowly, slept deeper and longer. The tension left my shoulders. "I guess we'll have to move to the ocean someday," he joked. Over the years, we've settled for regular visits, usually made in the cooler spring or fall—as a northwesterner, I prefer my coastline breezy and deserted. The beach is the only place where I know how it feels, even temporarily, to live without anxiety: I'm able to feel a kind of soul-deep calm I never get close to anywhere else.

It was the same for my mother; when she was a girl, it was her first glimpse of the ocean that planted a wish in her heart to live somewhere beautiful. If one or both of us were stressed, if we were getting into too many arguments or just feeling a little world-weary, she'd say, "Should we go to the coast this weekend?" and soon we'd find ourselves in the car, making the familiar drive through the mountain passes to the little fishing town my grandma and I had discovered one long-ago spring break. Until I was sixteen, we made free use of my grandparents' RV, parked in a trailer park a short drive or bike ride from the ocean. After Grandma sold it, Mom would manage to find money for gas and a couple of nights in the motel across from the marina. She and I would walk along the beach for miles, sometimes chatting, often silent, listening to the waves and hunting for sand dollars. These weekend trips were the only vacations she and I ever took together, but it didn't occur to me to wish for more: when you can get to the Pacific in under three hours, it's hard to feel anything but lucky.

With the anniversary of her death approaching, I can think of only one place where I might be able to weather it. I take the week off work, we tell the kids they can skip virtual school, and we find a house on the water where we can bring the dog. It's not the most beautiful beach I've been to—more bay than ocean, with a startling number of horseshoe crabs—but it's good to be there together, to introduce the dog to sand and cold salt water, to seek quiet and stillness instead of trying to work and push through our grief. The best feature of the house is a wide screened-in porch with lumpy old sofas, where we spend most of our time when we're not by the water. We play board games and read books; my kids draw; I write. Peggy's fur is always rumpled and damp, but she's happy. When we return from the beach, she naps long and deep, her head on my lap.

It is one year to the day since Mom died. We watch the sunset from borrowed beach chairs. She has been in my heart all week, so close I almost feel that I could speak to her and she would answer. I am still caught in the first wave of grief; I have no way of knowing what future tides will bring. I know that this is not pain without aim or form, even if it is pain without end. It is proof of how much I miss her, my love for her in another shape.

Beside my chair, our dog's paws drag at the sand; these are the first holes she has ever dug, and now digging is her vocation. My kids giggle at her industriousness, though it's clear that they are ready to no longer be sandy, to return to the house for showers and games and ice cream. As they begin rolling up their towels, folding up their chairs, I pull my phone out of my pocket and search for a poem I saved long ago: "What the Living Do," by Marie Howe.

I first encountered it when I was twenty-two, an age when I'd barely known grief, and was so moved by Howe's words that I kept the poem to reread and eventually bought all of her books. Addressed to her brother John, who died of complications from AIDS, "What the Living Do" has always seemed to me a perfect expression of love, and loss, and what it means to survive. It's been a few years since I last thought of it, but now that I need it, it's waiting for me, as the best poems do.

But there are moments, walking, when I catch a
glimpse of myself in the window glass,

say, the window of the corner video store, and I'm
gripped by a cherishing so deep

for my own blowing hair, chapped face, and
unbuttoned coat that I'm speechless:

I am living. I remember you.

How do you learn to cherish your life when grief has
made it unrecognizable? I am starting to feel that we do so
not by trying to fill a void that can never be filled but by living as best as we can in this strange, yawning terrain our
loved ones have left behind, exploring its jagged boundaries
and learning to see it as something new. I believe this because
I feel that I am becoming someone new—someone who can
remember, and mourn, and live without punishing herself.

My mother loved her life enough to fight for every last
moment, clinging to it with all her formidable will. Just as
fiercely as she wanted to live, I know that she wanted me to
have this life with my family, one that was always going to
go on without her, and to treasure it if I can. Not because it is
without fear or pain, loneliness or loss, but because it is mine.
It is a revelation to discover that I can be grateful, even glad
for it, though I will never stop missing her. I know that she
would consider this further proof of God's grace. I can only
think of it as a gift from her.

29

ON THE LAST DAY I GET TO SPEND WITH MY MOTHER, I don't know that it's the last day. I don't know that a virus is already spreading through the world, one that will upend our lives and rob us of what would have been our final visit. As her friends leave, taking paperwork to be notarized and lists of tasks to complete, I only know that I am lonely, afraid that my dying mother is angry with me. There is a part of me that remains a child, her child, searching for consolation I cannot find. I'll be spared the shock I experienced when Dad died, but this *knowing* is another kind of anguish—it is impossible to find comfort in the warning, the ability to see fresh grief bearing down on me.

Later, her priest arrives to pray with her and give her Communion, and I leave the two of them and go sit with my daughter in the spare room. I check my messages, text my husband to check in. I think about how Mom and I are having the unbearably hard but necessary conversations—

about end-of-life decisions, about her will, about treatment and hospice care—that we never got to have with Dad when he was alive. Maybe this is something to be grateful for, as wrenching as it is for both of us. I am not my father, I'm not her partner or her confidant, but I have had to grow into a new role as her daughter. I tell myself that we are both doing the best we can.

When the priest is ready to leave, I walk him out, mostly so I can ask him the question I have been turning over in my mind ever since my father's funeral. "You said that Dad knew he was dying," I say to him, shivering without a coat under my mother's carport. "You said he'd made his peace with it. How can you be so sure?"

"Your father and I talked, often, in his final months," he says. "He didn't *want* to die, to leave you or your mother. But he prepared himself. He forgave everyone, and he knew that he was forgiven. If he had known the exact day he would die, I don't think he would have done anything differently."

The thought is more comforting than it once was. What he describes is what I want for my mother—the kind of peace my father knew, if there is no way for her to have the long life she deserves. I want her to be able to prepare herself in whatever ways she can. I know how important her faith is to her, how much solace she stands to gain from it. I nod, hear myself thanking him.

When I go inside, I can see that the priest's brief visit has left my mother calmer, steadier. She's had enough of heavy business for the day and tells my daughter to fetch her jewelry boxes from her room. One by one, she shows her several pairs of earrings, lifting them out and holding them up to the light.

"Do you like these ones? They're amethysts, your birthstone," she says.

"They're pretty," my daughter, who has much simpler taste and avoids colors like purple and pink, says politely.

"Look, these are pearls. Your great-grandma gave them to me for Christmas one year."

I almost tell my mom that it's too soon to be giving us her things. But she's smiling, so happy to see my daughter try on a pair of small pearl studs. "These are all things I don't really wear anymore," she says, "so if you like them, you should take them now."

For me, she has a ring that her mother gave her: a large black oval of onyx inset with a small diamond. It's not a ring I ever asked to try on when I was a little girl; it wouldn't have drawn my eye then—it's not a sparkly or colorful jewel that a child would be drawn to, but a statement piece, dramatic and elegant. It is a ring, I think, that you have to grow into.

I slide it onto my right forefinger, the only one it fits, and think about the last time she gave me one of her family rings: a vintage ring she'd inherited from her aunt Mary, originally set with a row of three garnets and stacks of tiny pearls. It was a lovely thing, with delicate filigree scrollwork along the band, and as a child I thrilled to see it gleaming like a small crown on my finger. Mom would let me wear it for a few moments, never for long. "It's an heirloom," she said. "You'll get it when I'm gone." But on my twenty-fifth birthday, I received a package containing a photo album of my childhood and the ring I had long loved, nestled in a gray velvet box—cleaned, sized, and reset with deep purple amethysts in place of the old garnets. My mother didn't wait until she died to pass it on to me; instead, she freely gave me something she loved, something precious, long before the expected time.

When my daughter takes Buster out for his afternoon walk around the park, I take the opportunity to ask my mom about the ritual I witnessed earlier in the day, when each of her friends took her hands and asked her to forgive any of their offenses. In her church, she explains, Forgiveness Sunday marks the beginning of Lent. Parishioners take turns asking one another for forgiveness. No matter what may lie between two people, the only response is *I forgive you, and God forgives you.*

"Some people will ask one another for forgiveness all the time. You might do it when saying goodbye to someone who's ill, or traveling, or someone you might not see for a long time." Her voice brightens, infused with new energy despite how tired she is; this is how she always sounds when she's speaking about her faith, or her friends, or anything she loves. "I find it comforting to know that, if nothing else, at least I've forgiven people. It's necessary, and it works both ways: you don't want someone to not forgive you, and you don't want to forget to forgive someone else. You have to forgive for your own sake. Always make forgiveness part of your farewell."

There are tears in my eyes now, which I make no effort to hide as I sit beside her. "I hope you can forgive me for all my failures as a daughter."

"Forgive you?" She shakes her head. "There's nothing

to forgive, from where I am, but I forgive you everything. You did everything you could. You walked your path, you stayed faithful in your own way, and that's all I can ask. And who knows," she adds, "maybe, after I'm gone, we'll meet in prayer from time to time. Like the saints did."

I hold her as tight as I dare, both of us now weeping. It is the first time in weeks, months, maybe years, that I have felt more like her child than a parent. "This is your final battle, you know that. You should have gotten so much more time," I say. "But if you can't have that, then I want you to be able to feel some peace, and have time to prepare, the way Dad did."

"I told the priest that I'm afraid to die," she admits to me. "I'm so afraid to meet our Lord. I don't feel worthy. What have I ever really done?"

The answer couldn't be more obvious to me if it were written in the air before us, but I understand why she asks, because I know the feeling of unworthiness all too well. I have always felt as though I have something to prove: I have to do more, be *better*, to make other people's gifts and offerings worthwhile; to earn their care or justify their faith. I spent years trying to live up to the noble sacrifice I believed my birth parents had made, while also trying to be good enough for other people to love. I am *still* living as if the choices made by others—from my first parents giving me up, to my adoptive parents loving me and then letting me leave—are debts I have to repay, marks in a ledger I can never hope to expunge. Even this trip, and all the essential tasks I've assigned myself—have I not approached them as though I have something to atone for? As if there exists some list of things a good daughter does for her dying parent, responsibilities I didn't fulfill for my father, and now I have to prove my love and loyalty by ensuring that I don't fail again?

But my mother has never thought of my life or our relationship in such a way. Even when she has been upset with me, confused over decisions I've made, saddened by the physical distance between us, I have never had to do anything to prove myself to her. I am *enough* for her, without any action or justification, without proofs, just as I am. That's what she meant when she told me, as a child, that I could never disappoint her. That's why she and my father always said it didn't matter where I went, what I did with my life, what I accomplished—they would always be proud of me. That's why she believes that there is nothing for her to forgive now. I can choose to accept her at her word or not, keep chastising myself or not, but the truth is that this is what she has long believed: I am her daughter, so I am enough.

When she is gone, I wonder, can I possibly learn to be enough for myself? What would it mean—how would it feel—if I were?

She has asked me what she's done with her life, how she can stand before God without fear. I think again of my father, whom she'll soon be with, and how he might know what to say, how to reassure her, if he were here. But I am the person who is here now. My arms are the ones holding her, and I am the one who must try to give her an answer.

"You're a loving, good, and generous person," I tell her. "You've tried to live the life you thought God wanted for you. You've been the best mother to me. I'm so lucky to be your daughter."

It might not be enough for everyone, I know, at the end of their lives. But to me it has been everything. It is our life as parent and child, and I hope she believes in its value. I hope she knows that *she* was enough for me. This is all that is left to us—to hold and to love each other, to forgive, to grieve while we can.

She hugs me again, and says that we shouldn't be a mess when my daughter returns. We are sitting side by side on the sofa, holding hands, drying our eyes, when my daughter walks in with the dog. Mom announces that she's going to take a little nap before dinner and gets up carefully, gripping my hand for support. We walk down the hall together, Buster trailing behind us.

"You know," she says, before I leave her, "I can't seem to remember any of the bad times now that Dad is gone. I always think of him smiling or laughing or making some joke. I think of all the times when I was in a bad mood and he cheered me up. I only seem to remember the good times now."

"Because you loved him," I say.

I return to the living room and sit on the couch beside my daughter. In her expression I read compassion, sadness, weariness. A deep well of concern. Her face was the first I ever glimpsed that looked anything like mine—from the moment of her birth, I knew that I was not alone. Now nearly twelve, she never resembles me more than when her steady brown eyes, my eyes, are like this, serious and appraising. She has always been her own person, frequently leaving me, the person who birthed her, wondering where she came from and who she will be. And yet I know she is who she is in part because I am her mother, just as I am who I am because of mine.

"Mama," she says, "are you okay?"

I know she means in this moment, not all the ones to come. I reach for her, pull her into a hug, and give her the truth. "I'm not okay," I say. "But someday I will be."

I will be. Because of her, and her sister, and my husband, and everyone who loves me. Because my parents love me, and to live is to remember them.

I will always miss my mother. In the months and years to come, I'll wish for many impossible things: that cancer had never invaded her body; that the world had not changed; that I could be with her when she died; that I could have split myself in two, defied the laws of the universe and linear time, to be present in every moment she and my father needed me.

But I will also feel a deep and profound gratitude for our last day together. For whatever it was—love, grace, chance, or premonition—that pushed me to ask for her forgiveness, tell her that her life was a blessing and I was lucky to be hers. I won't have to wonder if she understood or forgave me. I'm not holding on to anything I wish I'd told her. In the end, there was nothing broken or left unsaid between us.

While my mother sleeps, my daughter and I sit side by side, our faces half-lit by the westward-facing windows, watching the sun creep down to the edge of the mountains my parents and I have known and loved in every season. We talk about the evening ahead: When Mom wakes up from her nap, we'll ask what she wants for dinner, burgers or tacos. Maybe we'll watch a movie, or play a game of cards—she is teaching my daughter how to play rummy—or maybe we'll just sit and talk until it's time for us to go to bed. We have to leave in the morning, but we still have one more night.

I keep my arm around my daughter, and together we wait for my mom to wake.

NOTES & ACKNOWLEDGMENTS

I AM DEEPLY GRATEFUL TO MARIE HOWE, WHOSE WORDS have long been a source of solace and inspiration, for permitting me to title this book with a phrase from her poem "For Three Days" and excerpt "What the Living Do" within.

The quotations from Saint John Climacus's *The Ladder of Divine Ascent* are from the 2012 Revised Edition by the Holy Transfiguration Monastery in Brookline, Massachusetts, translated by Father Lazarus Moore.

A Living Remedy exists thanks to the skill and abiding faith of Ecco publisher Helen Atsma, my editor and fellow Oregonian. From our first conversation, it was clear how much she believed in and understood this book, two things that remained true even as the story I thought I would write gave way to something new and far more arduous. Thank you, Helen, for helping to make this the book it needed to be, and for the abundant grace and care you've shown me.

Warmest gratitude to my agent, Maria Massie, source of so much compassionate advice, whose dedication and thoughtfulness has made all the difference in my career: how lucky I am to have you in my corner.

To Carrie Frye, who's had to listen to me talk about this book for longer than anyone else, and whom I was thrilled to collaborate with after years of trading editorial quips and metaphors: thank you for believing when I didn't, seeing what I couldn't, and not letting me go onstage with my kilt on my head.

I have the most brilliant and supportive publishing team, and am forever indebted to the all-star crew at Ecco Books, including Sonya Cheuse, Jin Soo Chun, Meghan Deans, Caitlin Mulrooney-Lyski, Miriam Parker, and Rachel Sargent. Many thanks to Michael Taeckens of Broadside PR. And Vivian Rowe, your cover is a dream—a poem in and of itself.

Heartfelt thanks to Julie Buntin, Kat Chow, Yuka Igarashi, Megha Majumdar, Imani Perry, and Bryan Washington for their generosity, care, and early reads. Jasmine Guillory, I treasure our friendship and genuinely don't know where I'd be without you. Crystal Hana Kim and R. O. Kwon, sisters and stalwarts of the group chat, I am thankful for you every day.

Much gratitude to Kristie Ahola, Angela Chen, Nicole Cliffe, Tope Fadiran, Alyssa Keiko Furukawa, Elon Green, Taylor Harris, Anna Hetherington, Danny Lavery, Karen Maeda Allman, Rita Maldonado, Rebecca Onion, Greg Pak, Samantha Powell, Chanda Prescod-Weinstein, Ingrid Rojas Contreras, Jaya Saxena, Christina Tucker, Esmé Weijun Wang, Maria Wheeler, and Jess Zimmerman. Tajja Isen, Matt Ortile, Stella Cabot Wilson, Allisen Hae Ji Lichtenstein, Leah Johnson, Arriel Vinson, Gabrielle Bellot, Eliza Harris, Sirin Thada: I'm always rooting for you.

I continue to be grateful for the ongoing efforts of Megan Fishmann and Lena Moses-Schmitt at Catapult and Elaine Trevorrow at EMT Agency. Thank you to all the booksellers and librarians and educators who have stocked or shared my books (special shoutout to Hannah, Christine, and Amy at Loyalty Books for setting up a signed preorder campaign in record time, during a week when half of us were on vacation!). And sincere thanks to all those who've spent any time with my writing over the years.

I want to acknowledge the compassion and labor of the many friends, health-care workers, hospice staff, therapists, and others who supported my family when we needed it most. I will never forget what you did for us.

All my love and gratitude to my parents, who gave me everything. To Cindy and Rick, who didn't have to but chose to be my family. To my daughters, heroes of the nineteenth and best generation. And to Dan, whose love and care has been the center of my life for over twenty years: None of this is possible without you. Thank you for being my harbor and my home.